BECOME A
FAT-BURNING MACHINE

THE 12-WEEK DIET

MIKE BERLAND
with GALE BERNHARDT

Regan Arts.
New York

Mike

*For my Argentine Princess,
who is the love of my life and my true north*

Gale

*For my husband, Delbert,
who is my rock of support*

CONTENTS

A SCIENTIFIC BREAKTHROUGH

The Fat-Burning Machine Diet Bridges
the Gap in Nutritional Thinking

By Stacy Sims, PhD

*Stanford University exercise physiologist–nutrition scientist
and cofounder of Osmo Nutrition*

I am very pleased that Mike and Gale have written this book. For years I have been talking about the divide between medical practitioners and nutrition scientists regarding how people should eat and exercise. With the Fat-Burning Machine Diet, Mike and Gale have bridged that divide. Mike's deep hunger for solutions and Gale's commonsense approach have produced a result that is consistent with the science I've found in my research at Stanford, the University of Otago, and my research consultancy, as well as in my athletes' and my own professional athletic endeavors.

The Fat-Burning Machine isn't just a clever turn of phrase; it's an actual description of how our bodies are designed to work. The plan incorporates nutrition and exercise in a synchronized way that is effective. The science is solid and people need to understand it, but there has been an absence of scientific discussion about these very important connections. One salient factor is that the medical community and the nutrition community are separately siloed in their own expertise. It's not really their fault. It's just the way they've been trained and organized. Most registered dietitians don't have a background in exercise physiology, so they don't always appreciate the connection between nutrition and exercise. Medical schools barely address exercise and nutrition; thus MDs and internists have very little background or expertise to counsel their patients on these matters. This silo effect leaves everyone narrowly focused—even though the science is suggesting a more holistic approach.

The end result is a lot of misinformation being disseminated to the public. Consider how the popular notions of what constitutes a healthy diet have come about. Back in the 1980s, there was a huge wave of opinion that a healthy diet should be low in fat and high in carbohydrates. Everyone got on the bandwagon, and the result was an obesity epidemic. As people replaced fat with sugar, America developed a major sweet tooth. Today everything has added sugar in it—even foods like bread, which shouldn't be sweet. Then the fitness industry got on board and told people they needed high-carbohydrate diets to perform in their workouts. And people were getting fat and experiencing many related health problems.

In current times, there has been a backlash to high-carbohydrate eating. That's why you're seeing diet trends such as the Paleo diet, which is very high in fat and low in carbohydrates. The problem is, the pendulum has swung too far in the other direction. It's based on a knee-jerk reaction to obesity, using a faulty reading of the science. In time, people will discover that this extreme diet approach doesn't work either—especially for women. It changes their hormonal activity in ways that increase fat storage and menstrual dysfunction. In short, extreme "fixes" don't work. They're a terrible disservice to people who really want a true pathway to wellness.

The appealing thing about the Fat-Burning Machine Diet, from a scientific perspective, is that it emphasizes clean, balanced eating— the right combinations of food from the best sources—that produces true health benefits. For example, looking at the list of fat-storing vs. fat-burning foods, the underlying fact is that the fat-"burning" foods are actually anti-inflammatory foods. With less systemic inflammation, the body is under less "stress," and is less inclined to store fat and create an environment for metabolic syndrome.

Your body is a machine, and this diet figures out how to keep it running as it's intended to run. Look at the results. On the Fat-Burning Machine Diet, your body produces less cortisol (aka the "belly fat hormone"). You have less inflammation. You're staying more hydrated. You have less central nervous system fatigue, so you can push harder and recover faster. Your skin and hair have more luster, and you're sleeping better. All of these benefits come together holistically to make you a generally healthier person.

> Fat-"burning" foods are actually anti-inflammatory foods. With less systemic inflammation, the body is under less "stress," and is less inclined to store fat.

The underlying story is about hormones. I find that many of the problems people have with diet and fitness begin popping up as they get into their forties. They've been cruising along on certain diet and exercise programs, and suddenly even those who have been fit find that the old go-to training and nutrition habits aren't producing the results they are used to. They start getting more abdominal fat, and they can't hit the same intensities in their workouts. Of course, they're very unhappy. But they don't realize that this isn't a sudden phenomenon. Those hormonal changes have been occurring under the radar for a long time.

We all know people in their twenties who have terrible diets but seem to get away with it. They say, "I have high metabolism," and everyone accepts it at face value. But when they don't see it overtly, there's an undercurrent going on—subtle hormonal responses to the food they're eating, their sleep patterns, their life stresses—as well as reproductive hormones that are not necessarily picked up on blood tests. People aren't usually aware of these changes because they're not overt. So they're surprised and unhappy when they get to their forties and they start noticing problems.

Men and women have different issues. For women, as their estrogen and progesterone levels and ratios change, long before menopause, they become sensitive to carbohydrates and they start gaining weight—specifically, putting on fat around the abdomen. For men, it's the gradual decline in muscle mass and the effects of declining testosterone. But while men and women have different hormonal impacts, they can find common ground in the program presented in this book.

It all comes back to the need for nutrition and exercise science to work together. While working in the Stanford Prevention Research Center (SPRC), the center of all research in physical activity and nutrition, it was very apparent to me that the physical activity research scientists were myopic in their expertise, and the nutrition research scientists were myopic in theirs: The physical activity scientists would factor nutrition as a cofounding variable, and the nutrition research scientists would put physical activity into an "afterthought variable" column. The integration of the two was a rarity, and for most, it didn't even cross their minds! When your physician is looking at how to treat metabolic syndrome, most of the research he or she is reading is about reducing carbohydrates, with little attention to the exercise component. The question never gets asked—how does physical activity mitigate the onset of metabolic syndrome? The best thing about the Fat-Burning Machine Diet is that nutrition and exercise work so beautifully in concert. It's the right path and an excellent example of how science can change the trajectory of your health, fitness, and life.

Many people are legitimately frustrated by the absence of practical information and support when addressing their weight and fitness issues. Often they've had negative experiences with popular diets that promised big but did not deliver. The Fat-Burning Machine Diet is a scientific approach for people at all levels of fitness. Remember, your body is designed to work this way. It's a real breakthrough to know you can give your body what it needs—and succeed.

Dr. Stacy Sims has contributed to the environmental exercise physiology and sports nutrition field for more than fifteen years as both an athlete and a scientist. Her personal interest in sex differences and performance has been the basis of her academic and consulting career—always looking at true physiology to apply innovative solutions in the sports nutrition world. Stacy served as an exercise physiologist and nutrition scientist at Stanford University from 2007 to 2012, specializing in sex differences of environmental and nutritional considerations for recovery and performance. Preceding her work at Stanford, she was a senior research scientist at Otago University, where she transferred her PhD work of sex differences in hydration and exercise in the heat to investigating the interactions of human performance, fabrics, and extreme environmental conditions. An elite athlete herself, Stacy has extensive experience working with athletes at the highest levels of sport worldwide, from the Olympics to the Tour de France.

THE FAT-BURNING MACHINE PROMISE

Nine Ways the Fat-Burning Machine Diet
Will Change Your Life

Congratulations. By opening this book, you are embarking on an important journey. Before we get started, I want to make a promise: The Fat-Burning Machine Diet will change your life in unexpected ways. It's not just about losing weight, although that will happen. It's not even just about achieving a higher level of fitness, although that will happen, too. The biggest surprise for people who go on this diet is that it improves their overall well-being. The checklist is impressive:

- Improved body shape

- Reduced belly fat

- Better tone in arms and legs

- Better sleep at night

- Better recovery from workouts

- Less food needed during workouts

- Reduced or eliminated hot flashes

In this book, we will show you how to optimize your performance so that your body looks and functions the way that you want. You'll discover a new sense of control. You'll *feel* better. There's a good reason people hate most diets. They feel lousy. They're hungry, moody, grouchy, foggy-brained, and just downright miserable. When I became a Fat-Burning Machine, my body got a much-needed tune-up and just started humming along. In fact, the most magical part of my journey was encountering all the extra benefits that I had never anticipated. Here are nine amazing benefits of the Fat-Burning Machine Diet:

1. IMMEDIATE WEIGHT LOSS

Everyone who goes on the Fat-Burning Machine Diet loses some weight right away. And the weight loss continues steadily. The people we've surveyed report losing at least one to two pounds a week, and some have had even greater results—six to ten pounds in the first three weeks of the diet.

Each person's body is different, but the results show one common thread: The weight loss begins to happen immediately. Susan's experience was typical. A self-described "yo-yo dieter" her entire life, she had reached her highest weight ever—241 pounds—when she started the Fat-Burning Machine Diet. Within 4 months she lost 27 pounds and 18 inches. Best of all, she did it without hunger cravings that had sabotaged previous diets. *The promise: You'll achieve fast and steady weight loss.*

2. LOOK TEN YEARS YOUNGER

People report looking younger on the Fat-Burning Machine Diet, and I can attest to that. Once I became a Fat-Burning Machine, the tone, feel, and tightness of my facial skin changed fairly quickly. I tend to gain weight in my face, which gives me a puffy, pale look. After I started the diet, my skin color became flush and it started to glow. My skin felt less dry and brittle. It was as if I was using a miracle moisturizer. My face quickly tightened up, and I no longer looked so puffy. My double chin disappeared. I lost ten years in less than ten months. Today I look younger than most of my friends. *The promise: Your skin will look and feel vibrant and younger.*

3. BOUNDLESS ENERGY

Tom, a surgeon who went on the Fat-Burning Machine Diet, knows how important it is to be alert and energized. In his line of work, it could be a matter of life and death! Within three weeks on the diet, he reported, "In a nutshell, I feel great, more alert, and have more sustained endurance through a day of long difficult cases and surgeries. I'm not famished midday or midafternoon anymore."

Greater energy throughout the day is one of the best things about this diet. I have always been an active person, but I now feel that I have limitless energy, and I enjoy everyday activities more. I take the stairs, and I enjoy walking and doing chores around the house. I no longer need to sit down a lot—I even have a standing desk. *Promise: You'll have more energy than ever for the everyday tasks and pleasures of life.*

4. SLEEP LIKE A BABY

People tend to underestimate the importance of a good night's sleep. If you don't sleep well, it has a domino effect on the rest of your day. Studies show that poor sleep also slows down your metabolism and makes it harder to burn fat. Poor diet habits upset your hormones and disrupt sleep.

I noticed the sleep benefit of the Fat-Burning Machine Diet very soon after I started. Falling asleep and staying asleep was always such an issue for me. I was such a restless sleeper. Now, I fall asleep quickly and sleep through the night in a deep, relaxed manner. In the morning I jump out of bed, ready to take on the day. *Promise: You'll sleep well and feel completely rested in the morning.*

5. AN END TO MOOD SWINGS

Mood swings are debilitating. And although they seem to be mental, they're actually physiological. When your body stores fat and doesn't process sugar properly, it affects your stress hormones and makes your moods feel like a roller coaster. I hated that side effect of being overweight more than anything else. I tend to be a happy and optimistic person, but the mood swings took over and made me anxious and nervous. I didn't feel like the "real" me. I am now calmer and more clearheaded. *Promise: You'll feel happier and less stressed.*

6. NO MORE HUNGER AND CRAVINGS

Nearly everyone who struggles with being overweight describes their biggest problem as food cravings—especially for sugar. I can relate. For most of my life I was a binge eater, and my binges were triggered by cravings I couldn't seem to control. On the Fat-Burning Machine Diet, not only am I satisfied with the food—no more hunger pangs!— but the cravings are gone.

People who have gone on the Fat-Burning Machine Diet report the same thing—especially what they experience as an "addiction" to sugar. As Lisa, one of our fat-burners, reported, "After five weeks on the program, I am more satisfied after meals; I don't have the sugar hunger cravings that plagued my diet. I really enjoy eating this way— my taste buds have changed, and I now enjoy much more flavor in all the foods I eat. This is a sustainable nutrition plan vs. a 'diet,' as I don't feel deprived." After eleven weeks, Greg was amazed at the results: "I have lost twenty-two pounds and lost four inches around my waist. I do not have the hunger cravings I was having before I cut out the sugars." *Promise: You'll feel satisfied and full.*

7. DIGESTIVE DISTRESS DISAPPEARS

When I was overweight, I developed acid reflux. It was horrible, and I started taking Prevacid to relieve the pain. Acid reflux isn't just uncomfortable. It creates a terrible cycle of health problems. Ultimately, my reflux resulted in two bouts of pneumonia within one year. Once I became a Fat-Burning Machine, my acid reflux went away and has never come back. Not one day. Diet participants report similar experiences with digestive distress, including no longer feeling sick after eating. *Promise: No more digestive agony.*

8. JOINTS STOP ACHING

One of my friends has a joke that goes something like, if you don't wake up aching, you are probably dead. Before I started the Fat-Burning Machine Diet, I was starting to think that was my reality. As I became heavier, I really felt my age. If I exercised or played a round of golf, I always suffered with creaky joints and pain in my knees and shoulders. And then suddenly, it all went away when I became a Fat-Burning Machine. The inflammation decreased, and I wake up ache-free every morning. My legs no longer feel like tree trunks after I exercise. *Promise: Fitness you can enjoy—no more aching joints.*

9. A FEELING OF WELL-BEING

The best thing about the Fat-Burning Machine Diet is that you'll feel healthier and more alive. Before the diet, I always seemed to have a cold or other flu-like symptoms—a cough, a sniffle, an ear infection, and a dull headache. Something always seemed to plague me. Those symptoms have all gone away. No sick days in the last four years!

Paul, who started the plan after seeing how well it worked for a friend, describes that wonderful feeling of well-being: "For me it has been a comprehensive lifesaving program that incorporates better eating and better exercise into my life. I wouldn't say it's a diet, or an exercise program, it is a new way to live your life. I am happy to report I've dropped almost 20 pounds in just under two months. I now weigh 176 pounds. My energy level is through the roof, and I'm experiencing far less back pain. In short, the path that the Fat-Burning

Machine program has put me on is a guide for the rest of my life. I can't believe I didn't do it sooner, and I'm never going back to that other way of living." *Promise: You'll discover a new sense of well-being.*

Who doesn't want to feel this way? And that's the promise of the Fat-Burning Machine Diet. Take the journey with us, and see for yourself. It will change your life. I promise.

PART ONE

FROM A FAT-STORING TO A FAT-BURNING MACHINE

ONE

I WAS A FAT-STORING MACHINE

Forty-plus Years of Heavy Diet and Exercise Left Me Tired and Fat

For most of the past forty-plus years, I was a fat-storing machine. Sometimes I was able to slow it down, but I was never able to turn it off completely. It has been one of my life struggles, and I never really understood why it was so hard to stop gaining weight. My body just seemed to want to store fat, rather than burn it.

I watched the fat build up around my waist over the years. Pound by pound, inch by inch. I didn't know how it happened. I weighed less than 200 pounds throughout high school, and then I never saw that number again. From the time I graduated in 1986 to 2012, I gained 53 pounds, going from 192 to 245 pounds. I didn't gain it all at once. I didn't even gain the "freshman 15." I gained the weight a pound or two a year for 26 years! Every few years I had a new set point—195, 200, 205, 210, 215, 220, 225, 230, 235, 240, 245, and so on. And each time I hit a new set point, it was hard to go back to the previous one. As I reached my fortieth birthday, I was suddenly thinking that 250 pounds or even 300 pounds was more of a possibility than 200 pounds.

It wasn't for lack of effort. I wanted to lose weight, but my goal kept eluding me. Over the years I had tried so many different things, but none seemed to work. I was a great *starter*. I did every diet and fitness program that came out. High carb, low carb. No meat, all meat. I did every diet for a while and then gave up when they stopped working. (In my pantry, I still have the bars and shakes to prove it.) I always had some initial success with diets, but I could only get back to my last milestone weight. I could never go backward to a previous set point. None of the diets I tried actually worked for more than a short time.

I'm not a cynic, but it seemed to me that the whole point of the diet industry was for the diet or program to have short-term impact rather than long-term success. They get you on a program, make you change your diet or even buy their food for a set amount of time, and then tell you to go back to your normal life. How could that possibly work in the long term? It's a clever way to make money, because people buy into the promise, and then blame *themselves*—not the diet— when they fail.

The real problem is that most diets just don't work. They are moments in time rather than sustainable change. They treat symptoms for a while, without ever addressing the core. We can lose weight from time to time by eating less, but that only slows the process down. We never really turn off our fat-storing machines; we just get them to idle for a while and then when they go back on, it seems like they're stronger than ever.

I know this for a fact because, like I said, I was a great starter of diets and training programs. I have at least two full shelves of diet books in my library. Multiple copies of several of them. And for many years I was the gym's best customer with top-level membership—all the bells and whistles. But then I only went two, maybe three times before I gave up or became too busy. Working out in a gym felt monotonous, and I simply never grew to have a routine.

Gym life wasn't for me, but I loved to compete. I was always athletic. I exercised and played sports at various levels of intensity. The thing is, it didn't seem to matter. I kept gaining weight. I never made sustained progress, and I had no idea why. It didn't make sense. I was committed. It was just that I would get to a certain point and then the progress stopped. It was like I could only peel back the first layer of fat, but never get more of it to disappear.

The fat always came right back. It would come back faster than I lost it, and I would even gain more than I had lost. The idea of being slender and fit seemed like a lofty and utterly unobtainable goal for me.

I wasn't alone. Most of the people that I know are pretty busy—working and playing hard. Many of us already exercise. We are the weekend warriors. We like to run, we play pick-up basketball, we ski, we enjoy riding our bikes or playing the occasional doubles tennis match with our spouses and friends. We coach our kids' soccer teams, and we dream of having a regular Saturday golf game someday. We enjoy yoga and even give Spin classes a whirl occasionally. Even the people I know who aren't especially athletic would like to find exercises that fit their abilities and schedule.

And yet, whether we exercise or not, few of us are really satisfied with our bodies. Most of us feel that we have a few extra pounds that we would like to lose. We see the fat in the mirror around our waists, on our hips, and on our chins. We feel the weight in the tight fit of our jeans. Who doesn't know the dread of putting on a shirt or sweater that we haven't worn in a while and feeling it straining at the seams?

As we get older, it seems like those few extra pounds become a lot of extra pounds. We didn't gain them all at once—it took some time. But they do add up and they don't go away. Maybe it doesn't feel that bad because it is happening to our friends, as well. Our waistlines increase while our hairlines decrease. It just seems like a function of age.

But those extra pounds really bother us. Not because we see ourselves as fat, but because we think those extra pounds are unfair. Why do some people get to eat whatever they want and never gain weight?

I wanted to be fit. I even started using the term "Fat-Burning Machine" to describe the process of efficient metabolism I aspired to. But my workouts weren't getting me there. I had just about resigned myself to the fact that I would be fat my entire life. I figured we each have our *things*, and this was mine. I was the fat guy who does lots of sports.

In 2010 I was at a tipping point. I was over 230 pounds, my cholesterol was too high, and I had over a 40-inch waist. My doctor wanted to put me on medication. I was quickly getting to the point of no return.

> If you had asked me at my fattest point, did I have a better chance of winning the lottery or becoming a Fat-Burning Machine, I would have quickly said winning the lottery.

If you had asked me at my fattest point, did I have a better chance of winning the lottery or becoming a Fat-Burning Machine, I would have quickly said winning the lottery. I had more control over winning the lottery. I could improve my odds by buying more tickets. And somebody always wins, so there was a chance my number would come up.

I felt I had *no* chance of becoming a Fat-Burning Machine. I was reading all of those books, trying all of the diet and fitness programs, trying to improve my odds, but nothing was working.

A WORD OF INTRODUCTION

By now you're wondering, who is this guy and why am I listening to him? So, before we go further, there a few things that you need to know about me.

I have been a political pollster and strategist for twenty-eight years. I spend a good part of my time asking people questions in surveys and analyzing what they say. I am optimistic by nature and as you can imagine, extremely outgoing. I don't fade into the shadows or end up in corners at parties. On the other hand, I am fairly serious and thoughtful. While not overly ideological, my opinions are well informed and fact-based.

But what being a pollster really means (and why it's important to this story) is that I am interested in people and what motivates and persuades them. I like to understand what they do and why they do it and how I can change their attitudes or behaviors. I have also taken those skills that I learned on the campaign trail for candidates such as Hillary Clinton and former New York City mayor Michael Bloomberg and brought them into boardrooms for clients such as Facebook, BlackBerry, and the National Hockey League.

Working with some of the most interesting and successful people in the world, I became curious about how they achieved their success. I even collected their stories in my first book, *What Makes You Tick? How Successful People Do It and What You Can Learn from Them*. I fundamentally believe that successful people have secrets that they haven't yet shared about their achievements. Over the years, my inspiration, creativity, and curiosity came from so many different sources in the political, entertainment, and business world. I interviewed everyone from Heidi Klum to Bob Costas to Steve Forbes. Understanding the prototypes of success was a journey of self-learning for me. It helped me understand my own success, and I was happy to share their stories with others so that they could succeed as well.

I also get a lot of inspiration at home. I have been married for half my life. Literally. I am forty-seven, and I got married at twenty-three. My wife, Marcela, is from Argentina, and she is smart, confident, and beautiful. We met at work, and she is also a pollster, working for heads of state in Latin America. We have two incredible kids— Matthew, 21, and Isabella, 19. Marcela is one of those perfect people I described earlier—she has no weight issues and is probably in better shape today than when we got married. I used to think she was just lucky, but you know what? I was wrong. She works at it constantly. She is a Fat-Burning Machine and I never realized it. Why? Because I didn't know her secrets.

As a pollster, I am trained to look for patterns. I look for patterns in how people think and how they behave. I believe that everything is predictable and everything can be explained. I am more surprised when things don't happen the way that I expected than when they do.

I predict outcomes, based on varying sets of factors. Time and again, I have witnessed the ways people change their minds and behaviors when they receive new information. Maybe that's why I believed that I could find the answer to my questions. I wasn't satisfied with just being overweight. I figured that if I just asked enough people, I would find the solution to my problem. I believe in people. People have answers. I just had to ask the right questions.

A FINAL WAKE-UP CALL

For a long time I had been working toward competing in the Chicago Triathlon—in my old hometown. In 2010, I thought I was finally ready. I looked forward to the beautiful swim in Lake Michigan, the brisk ride up and down Lake Shore Drive, and a nice run past Soldier Field and McCormick Place into Grant Park. It was going to be a great way to see the old neighborhood.

This particular year it was *hot*. And when I say hot, I mean searing Chicago sun, sweltering 100 percent humidity, and oppressive heat. It was one of those days I remember from growing up in Chicago—when they'd warn the sick and elderly to stay indoors. Blistering.

I did the swim with no problem—I was a swimmer in high school—and even Lake Michigan was warm that day. The bike ride was spectacular, although I felt a little slower than normal. And then two miles into the run, I hit a wall like I have never done before. Everything just went into slow motion. My legs, my arms, my whole body just slowed down. I kept telling myself I would walk until the next water station and then I would start running again. It never happened. It took me one hour and forty-three minutes to complete six miles. It should have taken me an hour. And I felt beat.

It wasn't the first warning sign, but for some reason that experience was a big wake-up call for me. It was now or never. I had to do something about my weight and overall health. But how would I do it? I couldn't go on another diet. I couldn't endure another yo-yo effect. I needed real change or I would be 250 pounds before I knew it and my dreams of triathlons would fade away and so would my fitness. Something had to change—but what?

I knew if I was going to lose the weight this time, I would have to do things differently. During the 2008 presidential election, I remember sitting in the back of a campaign bus with Hillary Clinton on a cold dark night in Columbus, Ohio, after a campaign rally. By that point, Hillary was frustrated with how the race was going. She was exhausted and she said to me in an exasperated tone, "Why don't the voters get it? You don't hope for change. Change takes hard work." Those words have stuck with me for years, and I realized that if I was going to get the change that I wanted, I was going to have to work hard for it. I couldn't just buy the books, start the diet, or join the gym. I had to work harder. But more than that, I had to work *different*.

> I knew if I was going to lose the weight this time, I would have to do things differently. But how?

TWO

A FAT-BURNING SECRET REVEALED

The First Step to Understanding Why I Was Gaining Weight

After the Chicago Triathlon, I was miserable, lost in my thoughts, feeling like my weight was out of control. And then I got lucky when my friend Stu led me to Dr. Laura Lefkowitz. The introduction was made by pure happenstance. Stu and I are golf buddies and we were playing golf at Friar's Head, one of my favorite courses on Long Island.

I noticed that Stu looked absolutely amazing. Like me, he lived an active lifestyle but had a few extra pounds to lose. And he had lost most of them—over twenty pounds—since the last time I saw him earlier that summer. How had he done it? I was proud of him, but also jealous of his success.

I couldn't help myself. On the first hole, before he was able to even take his first putt, I began to quiz him. He told me that he had started seeing a cool nutritionist who had made weight loss easy for him. She had a magic combination of meals that made it easy to lose weight and not be hungry at all. Needless to say, I was interested and I scheduled an appointment with Dr. Lefkowitz as soon as I could.

That's how I found myself walking into a building in a Manhattan neighborhood somewhere south of Union Square and north of Greenwich Village.

Dr. Lefkowitz's office was spartan, and I saw immediately that this wasn't about fancy decor or pretense. No poseurs in this practice. Just people who wanted to get down and do the work necessary to lose weight. I was intrigued, but highly skeptical due to my past disappointments, and I took it out on the warm, attractive woman sitting across the desk from me.

As we started our conversation, I didn't make it easy for Dr. Lefkowitz. I peppered her with questions:

- What was different about her approach? I had tried every diet and followed every program in the past with fleeting results. I was past gimmicky stuff like Atkins or trendy diets like South Beach. I needed something deeper that I could get into and commit to for a longer period of time. I had also witnessed firsthand the failure of trendy surgeries like lap bands and staples. My mother had bariatric surgery around 10 years ago and instead of losing weight, she became masterful at beating the restriction or taking out the saline solution to loosen it. She developed severe acid reflux as well. I just didn't want to take a chance that would happen to me. I would rather be overweight and happy than have to endure that type of torture.

- How did I know that it would work? I realized there were no guarantees, but I didn't want to waste my time. I believe in the predictability of data. Who were Dr. Lefkowitz's other patients? Men? Women? Young? Old? How much did they have to lose? How did they do? Did they lose it? Did they keep it off? I had no desire to start drinking fitness shakes or meal replacements. I wanted real food that I could prepare at home and eat at restaurants. I also wasn't interested in a program that was designed to keep Victoria's Secret models thin. I didn't want to suddenly start eating air as my main course. I needed to know that Dr. Lefkowitz had patients like me.

- How long would it take? I really didn't know how patient I would be (no pun intended). The longer it took, the more frustrated I would be and the more likely I would be to drop it. On the other hand, I didn't want another short-term fix that didn't provide a long-term solution. I had to get my head in the game. So I would need to see steady results to keep the momentum and interest.

- Why was Dr. Lefkowitz qualified? I believe in insights. I expected her to know something or see something that others did not. I was looking for an unusual intuition or area of expertise that made her uniquely qualified to help me. Run-of-the-mill trainers, specialists in exercise, and nutritionists wouldn't work for me. I was completely convinced that there was something more interesting or scientific out there that I could tap into that would help me.

Dr. Lefkowitz was patient with me. She could feel my frustration, and she let me know it. She had a wonderful quality of empathy that began to put me at ease.

She answered my questions, but more importantly she made me curious to learn more. You see, Dr. Lefkowitz is a special type of nutritionist. She's an MD, with a deep understanding of body chemistry. Perhaps most comforting to me, Dr. Lefkowitz had once been fat herself. It was one of the factors that motivated her to choose a nutritional expertise. I could tell by looking at her that she'd found an answer for herself. And I liked the fact that she understood what it was like to struggle with weight. She wasn't going to preach or have me do something that she hadn't done herself.

That was a relief. As we talked, I relaxed.

Before our initial consultation, I'd filled out a long questionnaire, and now we talked about my answers.

There was one "catchall" question at the end of the questionnaire that struck me. Usually I would leave those blank, but this one I answered. It asked, "Anything else you would like to share?" And that was the moment of truth. Would I really share something that I had never told anyone else? Would I take a chance? I felt that I had nothing to lose, so I took the first step on my journey and acknowledged that I had a problem. I wrote that I felt like I was a compulsive binge eater. I ate when I was nervous or overworked or tired.

As we talked about my answers, I found that the feelings I'd kept bottled up for years started pouring out. I knew I was a fat-storing machine, but I couldn't stop.

Finally, Dr. Lefkowitz looked me straight in the eye and said, "Mike, this isn't so hard, and you don't have to be so emotional. You have a very common phenomenon. Many people share your problem."

But it felt emotional, not physical. Little did I know how wrong I was.

It was completely physical. And every day I was making it worse.

THE BIG BREAKTHROUGH

Before my visit, Dr. Lefkowitz had asked me to get a blood test to understand my cholesterol and blood sugar levels, telling me that the results would offer clues I could use. Now she turned to the facts.

She told me to look at my symptoms:

- I had been steadily gaining weight

- My waistline was increasing each year

- My cholesterol had been steadily rising

So, what did that mean?

Dr. Lefkowitz told me I had a textbook case of metabolic syndrome. I had to manage insulin and cortisol better, address my cholesterol problem, and lower my blood sugar. Left untreated, I was at significant risk for type 2 diabetes.

My mind was racing. Suddenly I was speechless. Excuse me? Metabolic what? Metabolic syndrome? Never heard of it. I mean, truly never heard of it. I have probably read and heard of everything else under the sun that had to do with being overweight. I hadn't heard of this one. Who even knew metabolic syndrome existed and that it was relevant to people with active lifestyles like me? I didn't. How could I suffer from metabolic syndrome? I wasn't one of those inactive people on the edge of serious health ailments. I wasn't prediabetic . . . was I? Nobody had told me about metabolic syndrome.

It was exactly the insight that I was looking for. I leaned forward in my chair. I wanted to learn.

Dr. Lefkowitz explained that metabolic syndrome was relatively new as far as syndromes are concerned. In fact, metabolic syndrome has only been diagnosed in the last twenty years, and yet it is as widespread as pimples and the common cold. According to the American Heart Association, forty-seven million Americans have it. The syndrome runs in families, and the risk of developing metabolic syndrome increases as you age.

Interestingly, metabolic syndrome is not a disease. It is a constellation of obesity-related factors that come together to make you a fat-storing machine.

You can't contract metabolic syndrome in an instant—it takes time—and in the same way, you can't really get rid of it so quickly. You can only control it.

I certainly fit the profile. But what I found so fascinating was that I knew I had some of those factors individually, but I had never really thought about them together. At my last physical, my primary doctor wanted me to start taking cholesterol medicine because my LDL (low-density lipoprotein—the "bad" cholesterol) had finally passed the normal threshold, and she'd suggested that I change my diet to start eating more vegetables, and maybe exercise a little more. Same old, same old. I saw now that my doctor was treating my symptoms, but she did not identify or treat my actual syndrome.

My mind traveled back to all the doctors I'd seen over the past twenty-five years. I couldn't think of a time I hadn't heard some variation of the standard advice: 1) Eat more vegetables, less French fries.

2) Try to exercise more. 3) Drink more water. It all started to sound like a Charlie Brown cartoon, "Waaa . . . waaaa . . . waaa." White noise.

But now, suddenly, with the diagnosis of metabolic syndrome, I got it. My weight gain was finally making sense to me. Not only was I overweight, but with metabolic syndrome, I was also at risk for heart attacks, strokes, and type 2 diabetes.

> My weight gain was finally making sense to me. Not only was I overweight, but with metabolic syndrome, I was also at risk for heart attacks, strokes, and type 2 diabetes.

Fortunately, metabolic syndrome was Dr. Lefkowitz's specialty. She could see it, diagnose it, and treat it like a pediatrician would treat a child's cold. And she was going to help me.

DR. LEFKOWITZ EXPLAINS METABOLIC SYNDROME

Dr. Lefkowitz explained to me that my symptoms and blood tests told the tale of my metabolic syndrome:

- High blood pressure
- High blood sugar
- Unhealthy cholesterol levels
- High triglycerides
- Excess abdominal fat

Metabolic syndrome is characterized as having three of the five symptoms listed above. Weight gain is only part of the picture. It's a very common condition. Statistics are my business, and this was a doozy: Health studies by the National Institutes of Health and the American Heart Association show that one-third of all Americans are affected by it.

Simply put, metabolic syndrome is a disorder that causes calories to be stored instead of burned. If you have metabolic syndrome, you're not good at using calories from sugar for energy. It's called insulin resistance. Insulin is a hormone that shuttles glucose into cells to be used as energy. The insulin receptors on your muscles operate under a lock and key system. The insulin docks in an insulin receptor, turns the key, and lets the sugar into the muscle. But when you have insulin resistance, the insulin doesn't open the door. You literally can't get sugar into the muscle.

When the sugar is locked out, it shuttles to the liver and is converted to stored fat. Other types of food like protein and fat are not dependent on insulin for providing energy. They go through different pathways, so you don't get the same effect. But sugar utilization—and that means carbs, especially simple carbs—is stymied. The fuel you think you're using for energy isn't working. It's like being a diesel engine and trying to run on regular gasoline.

> Insulin resistance is like being a diesel engine and trying to run on regular gasoline.

She also explained why exercise didn't stop my weight gain or food cravings. If someone has metabolic syndrome, they can't utilize calories well. Exercise is important for addressing metabolic syndrome, but if your fat-burning mechanism is blocked, you can still gain weight—even with exercise. And in addition to weight gain, there are other issues that interfere with your well-being—like fatigue, mood swings, and a general feeling that it's hard to get through the day.

Some experts estimate that even people who don't have more than one or two of the symptoms—and might not technically have metabolic syndrome—may be storing fat as a result.

- **Large waist circumference.** Sometimes called abdominal obesity, this is defined as a waistline that measures at least 35 inches for women and 37.5 inches for men. People who store fat around their waist are at much higher risk for diabetes, heart conditions, and obesity because that fat is hormonally active and prone to cause systemic havoc. If you have a large waist circumference, it's a sure sign that your body is storing fat.

- **High triglyceride level.** Triglycerides are a type of fat found in your blood. This is fat that is meant to be stored. If you eat more calories than your body needs, they get stocked away in your fat cells for later use. Over time, if you eat more calories than you burn, your triglyceride level goes up. High triglycerides are over 150 milligrams per deciliter (mg/dL)—meaning you're storing more fat than you're burning. Ideal triglyceride levels are under 100 mg/dL.

- **Reduced HDL cholesterol.** HDL is often referred to as the "good" cholesterol. LDL cholesterol is considered the "bad" cholesterol because it contributes to plaque, a deposit that can clog arteries. HDL cholesterol is considered "good" cholesterol because it helps remove LDL cholesterol from the arteries. It's good for heart health and keeps your engine running. Low HDL is less than 50 mg/dL.

- **Increased blood pressure.** Not only is this unhealthy, but studies show that being overweight goes hand in hand with high blood pressure. This condition is met if you are taking blood pressure medications or if your blood pressure is greater than 120/80 millimeters of mercury (mm Hg) at rest.

- **Elevated blood sugar.** Elevated blood sugar is a result of insulin resistance, when the cells are no longer sensitive to insulin. As a result, higher levels of insulin are needed in order for insulin to have its proper effects. So the pancreas compensates by trying to produce more insulin. Count this trait if you have a fasting blood sugar level above 100 mg/dL.

This list seemed daunting at first, but Dr. Lefkowitz assured me that even people with metabolic syndrome can beat the fat-storing cycle, lose weight, and achieve fitness. Best of all, we don't have to be hungry or miserable. The lifestyle changes that address metabolic syndrome also help people feel better and more energetic. For me, understanding metabolic syndrome was like opening a window and breathing fresh air.

> Metabolic syndrome is a disorder that causes calories to be stored instead of burned. If you have metabolic syndrome, you're not good at using calories from sugar for energy. Instead, they get stored as fat.

Dr. Lefkowitz also showed me that some clues could be found in my childhood. Not surprisingly, I was an overweight kid. It was enough of an issue that my parents and I knew that I needed to go on a diet when I was about ten years old. I was pretty independent and hard to control. So one day they came up with this brilliant idea that they'd help tame my eating impulses by locking the kitchen cabinets and refrigerator with chains. As I look back, I remember that it was quite embarrassing for me, but as I think about it more deeply, I realize that it was even more embarrassing for my parents.

It wasn't just the locks that got to me. As Dr. Lefkowitz explained, they were actually training my palate with the wrong kinds of food—especially so-called "diet" foods in portions too small to satisfy my hunger. Deprived of my many snacks, I lost weight, but it set me up for later failure—a lock-the-cupboards mind-set. I entered adulthood with a lot of baggage.

Now that I controlled the kitchen, I wasn't going to lock the cabinets—in reality or even metaphorically. Dr. Lefkowitz smiled and assured me that neither would she. She also told me something I found quite profound. My metabolic syndrome wasn't so much about simple genetics (which I'd always believed) as it was about history. She said, "If your mother had raised you on vegetables with exercise, and didn't lock those cabinets, you might have had a different relationship with food. But the relationship you had with food led you to overeating, binge eating, and gaining weight—and once you gained a certain amount of weight, you triggered insulin resistance."

Insulin resistance, the crown jewel of metabolic syndrome, was an idea I could get my head around. The scientific logic was impeccable. My cells were not using insulin for energy. Instead, the insulin was being stored as fat. In other words, my cells were locked just like those cabinets had been. And Dr. Lefkowitz was going to hand me the key.

BEATING METABOLIC SYNDROME

Dr. Lefkowitz and I spent the next nine months redesigning the way I ate. I found that if I wanted results, I had to change my current habits on a long-term basis. If I kept switching my Fat-Burning Machine on and off, I would only continue to gain weight and lose fitness.

In the past, I had inadvertently set myself up for failure. I didn't know that by eating the wrong foods, I not only was turning off fat burning, I was turning on my hunger hormone. I was exercising on a regular basis, but my routine was actually making me hungrier than when I started.

> I found that if I wanted results, I had to change my current habits on a long-term basis. If I kept switching my Fat-Burning Machine off (by eating foods that raised my insulin and cortisol levels), I would only continue to gain weight and lose fitness.

I could only end my vicious cycle by making changes. My old habits were killing me. Literally. I had to plan and prepare for my success every day. As I worked with Dr. Lefkowitz, I watched my weight drop from a high of 245 pounds to a low of 177 pounds.

I loved my new fitness. My waist shrunk down to a size 32. I had to buy a whole new wardrobe. It felt great. I went from extra-large T-shirts and sometimes extra-extra-large to size medium. I was suddenly the same size as my twenty-one-year-old son. What an accomplishment; a lifetime of extra weight gone in a matter of months. I felt giddy with success.

But not so fast. It turned out I still had more secrets to learn.

WHAT'S HAPPENING HERE?

Like most people, I have a bucket list. Nothing too crazy, all within reason, but a few were harder to achieve than others. Some of the items on my bucket list were personal achievement, some professional achievement, some fitness goals, and some family aspirations.

There were three things on my bucket list that I had virtually written off, but with my new fitness, I thought I should revisit them.

Mike's bucket list:

1. **Get under 200 pounds:** It had been twenty-five-plus years since I had seen this milestone, and I had already achieved it. Wow. Thanks, Dr. Lefkowitz.

2. **Run the New York City Marathon:** When I first moved to New York, the marathon went right past my apartment on First Avenue. What an amazing achievement it would be. I had actually signed up several times and even gained entry, but always had to defer because I was not in good enough shape to do the race.

3. **Complete the Ironman Triathlon in Kona, Hawaii:** Since my first triathlon in 1984, I had dreamed of racing the Ironman Championship through the lava fields in Hawaii. I watched the race broadcast and subscribed to *Triathlete* magazine.

I had achieved the first goal, almost effortlessly. Once I turned off my fat-storing machine, the weight melted away.

So I decided to be more ambitious and to try to knock another item off my bucket list. I wasn't going to be satisfied just running the Chicago Triathlon. I wanted to push the limits and go for more. This was the year that I was going to do the New York City Marathon. I had achieved my weight goal; now it was time to try to achieve some of my fitness goals.

I had never really gone more than 10K. My training runs for triathlons were between three and six miles. So the idea of going 26.2 miles was exciting and scary—way beyond anything I once thought was possible. I thought the training would be an excellent way to keep my Fat-Burning Machine running to its maximum and maintain my fitness.

I had no idea how to train for a marathon, and I had heard the horror stories—long, boring runs, achy knees, bleeding nipples. Yuck. I needed this to be fun and challenging. I needed a marathon coach. That's what led me to Coach Mike.

Coach Mike was my type of guy. He was a competitive marathoner, USA Track & Field Level 1 Coach, and coach of the Columbia University track team. He ran his own classes in Central Park, and he coached people with a wide range of abilities.

What I didn't know when I started marathon training is that Coach Mike is the King of Central Park. He has been running in the park for more than twenty years and has trained a good number of the runners who do their daily workouts in the park. They all know him and greet him as they pass by. It felt like I was training with royalty. Coach Mike is also distinctive because he doesn't have a left arm and can't be bothered wearing an artificial limb that is either cumbersome or uncomfortable. I was just in awe of how cool he is. I couldn't wait for my runs with him.

Coach Mike and I did workouts once a week, and on the other days he sent me workouts to do on my own. Some days it was distance workouts, other days it was accelerations. I could slowly feel my endurance and fitness building. Coach Mike trains by time, not by distance. I started doing 30-minute runs, 45 minutes, 115, 145, and 215, all the way up to three-hour runs. I was burning so many calories; I thought that keeping my weight down would be a breeze.

But it wasn't. To my shock, as I increased my distance, I was struggling to keep my weight down. In fact, the longer I went, the more weight I was gaining. *What was going on here?* It didn't make sense. Who has ever seen a fat runner? But that was what I was becoming. The more I trained, the more I gained. To say I was devastated is an understatement.

I was really struggling to figure out what was happening. I didn't think it was my diet. I was still following Dr. Lefkowitz's plans. I was eating the right combinations of food and I wasn't cheating. The only difference was that I was going longer distances and needed more energy to sustain my pace. When I was training for the Chicago Triathlons, most of my workouts had been less than an hour, other than an occasional bike ride of ninety minutes. For the twelve weeks leading up to the New York City Marathon, all my workouts were over an hour. And for the last eight weeks, most of my long workouts were over two hours.

I told Coach Mike that after about seventy-five minutes, I felt weak and shaky. He said that it was normal and that I should bring "goos" or "gels" to give me energy while I was running. He also said that I should consume sports drinks along with water when I was thirsty. This seemed like a good idea to me. Many runners were doing the same thing, and it made sense from what I was reading. My endurance was increasing as I was easily doing ten-, twelve-, fifteen-mile runs. I was achieving levels I had never had before. But my weight was steadily increasing. I couldn't stop gaining weight if I wanted to keep up the training.

Yet, despite the weight gain, I was ready to run the marathon. I had done my final twenty-three-mile run easily. I was beginning to do the advised tapering off before the marathon. And then Hurricane Sandy hit. After training all summer and dreaming about the NYC

Marathon for my whole life, I was going to have to put my dream on hold. New York was washed out, and many people didn't have electricity or heat. Instead of running over the Verrazano Bridge in Staten Island to start the marathon, my family and I went to Staten Island on the Saturday before the marathon and distributed fresh water, food, and canned goods. Our neighbors were in need, and we were there to help.

But it meant deferring my dream for another year. From my experience in 2012, I knew I could train and finish the marathon, but it would be another full year of training. An incredible effort. It was kind of like doing the marathon two years in a row.

But the marathon was on my bucket list and I was determined. So I started training with Coach Mike again. We did the same program, I ate the same gels and goos, and I gained the same weight. I was so happy to finish but so frustrated with the weight gain. Why did I have to sacrifice one for the other?

In 2013, I achieved my goal and finished the marathon. It was amazing. Five boroughs. Cheering crowds. I was so proud of knocking it off my bucket list—and also happy to never do it again. Once was enough for me. And I was slow. Even though in my head I wanted to go faster, I couldn't get my legs to cooperate. I ended up with a time of five hours and thirteen minutes, which was forty-five minutes slower than I expected.

> I was scared. Was I going to gain weight again? I was not able to drop all of the seven to ten pounds the first time. Would I gain even more? Was I going to go over 200 pounds?

But then it hit me—the bad news. Training for the NYC Marathon had turned off my ability to burn fat and keep my weight in check. I had been running my Fat-Burning Machine so efficiently for those nine months when I lost all the weight. What happened? I had become a fat-storing machine again. I couldn't believe it. I was lucky that I didn't gain even more weight. Was this the end? Was I going to be fat again?

It just didn't make sense to me, and so I began my quest for more answers. Somehow I mustered the determination not to give up. Dr. Lefkowitz had introduced me to a big fat-burning secret, but there were more secrets out there and I was determined to find them. And to make it even more of a challenge, Dr. Lefkowitz had closed her New York office and moved to Florida. I was on my own.

After gaining ten pounds training for the New York City Marathon, I was stuck, unable to lose the weight I'd gained. I was back to fat storing. During the marathon, I was exercising more than I had ever done in my life and my weight was steadily going up.

Would I have to write off my bucket list as unobtainable? If I gained any more weight, I was going to go over 200 pounds. Was it worth losing one bucket-list item for another? Not for me. Staying under 200 was a lifetime goal that I wasn't willing to give up. What bothered me most was that it just didn't make sense. The data did not compute. I needed to find out why.

However, my search for answers among the "experts" was less than enlightening. One of them suggested that I try to do shorter races faster. If I did do longer races, it would have to be a lumbering pace. The message was that people like me couldn't be fit and also perform. I was completely discouraged. I took a year off and golfed a lot, scheduling one or two games during the week and four games on the weekend—thirty-six holes each day. I walked the courses, carrying my clubs, playing in every tournament that I could find. But golf wasn't enough for me. I wanted more. I couldn't accept that striving to be an Ironman would make me fat again.

That's when I made a decision that changed my life. I sought out Gale Bernhardt. Gale is a former Olympic Triathlon team coach. She is truly one of the pioneers and gurus of triathlon training. Her training books are the bible of the sport, and her blogs are legendary. And since training was a big part of my life, even when I wasn't so successful, I was the guy on Active.com who bought Gale Bernhardt's training program each year. If her training programs were good enough for Olympians, they were good enough for me! So every day I received an email of a workout for that day. Gale's training programs just seemed like they were written specifically for me.

Gale brings out the best in everyone. She understands the goals and objectives and designs programs that work by combining training and nutrition. She understands the science and how the body works. Gale is curious and always looking for the next challenge. I was elated when she agreed to take me on as a client, and it turned out to be the best investment I've ever made.

I told Gale everything: my metabolic syndrome diagnosis from Dr. Lefkowitz and how I had lost sixty pounds. I described running the New York City Marathon with the help of Coach Mike. And, finally, I described my disappointment when I gained weight. I was exercising long and slow. Why wasn't it working?

Gale's formula would end up being simple, unconventional, and dramatic—a way to teach my body to stop storing fat and start burning it.

THREE

THE BURN EQUATION

Miracle Intervals + High-octane Foods

Before I met Gale, I'd always had a very clear mental picture of what it means to "burn" fat. I imagined one of those old-fashioned stoves, stoked with heavy shovels full of coal. The coal would incinerate, turn deep red, and then dissolve into ash. I thought burning fat on my body worked somewhat the same way. That's why I tortured myself with killer regimens. If sweat was pouring off my body, I was burning fat. Wrong, said Gale. "You think you're igniting your fat-burner. You're really cooling it off." What a revelation!

IGNITING THE FAT BURNER

It turns out that the conventional wisdom of long, sweat-pouring workouts being the best way to manage weight loss and metabolic syndrome is dead wrong. Burning fat actually requires mixing it up.

Exercising fast does not burn fat or improve your condition. As Gale taught me, when people train fast all the time, they end up averaging out to a sluggish speed. Strength deteriorates. Arms and legs get jittery. Breathing is labored. Meanwhile, on the inside, the fat-storing mechanisms are cranked to full gear. Very high exercise intensity, for periods over a minute or so, with very little rest actually turns off fat-burning. Visualize a group of people flogging themselves to exhaustion in an exercise class, with thought bubbles of *"More is better!"* and *"Go harder!"* floating above their heads.

It is actually best if very high-intensity exercise is combined with generous rest before the next interval. Lower levels of intensity can be combined with bouts of less rest to optimize fitness gains. It is all about level of intensity combined with appropriate recovery that aids in fitness gains. Too often exercisers go too "hard" for too long, thinking that if some intensity is good, then more and harder must be better. No pain, no gain was the motto that was burned into my brain. Wow, was that wrong!

Gale opened my mind to a new way of viewing fat-burning exercise that blew me away. She explained that a growing stack of studies, coupled with her own experience, show that interval training—which alternates a relaxed pace with bursts of high-intensity movement—generates better glucose control than steady-state cardio. Why? The intense contractions that fatigue muscles also break down carbohydrate stores in muscle. The muscles then become much more responsive to insulin as they attempt to replenish these stores. In fact, resistance training offers a bonus: It creates more muscle tissue and insulin receptors, further improving the absorption of glucose into muscles. They soak it up like a sponge. And muscle tissue is where glucose should be, not floating in your blood or being converted into fat. As the muscle absorbs all that glucose, the pancreas can breathe a giant sigh of relief. So the key is proper progression and not rushing into it too soon.

This is especially important for people who are out of shape, deconditioned, or already at the level of insulin resistance, diabetes, or cardiovascular disease. Studies show that moderate intensity seems to be more effective than low and high intensity when it comes to maintaining the insulin cell function. But the formula works for athletes at all levels. Everything I'd learned for the previous forty years was simply wrong.

THE MIRACLE INTERVALS

Gale had been experimenting with Miracle Intervals for several years when I met her. At the time, conventional wisdom favored long, steady efforts, but Gale had discovered a different method involving short intervals at high power output with very long recoveries. By using these intervals with cyclists, triathletes, and runners, she found that power and speed improved significantly, without long, torturous interval sets. She thought the method would be perfect for me because it wouldn't trigger my insulin resistance and may help me burn fat.

The basic routine was all-out power intervals lasting forty-five seconds or less with an easy recovery of four and a half minutes. At first it felt very strange to me. Remember, I was the all-out "no pain, no gain" guy. But those huge rest intervals actually generated tremendous output. I was performing better than ever. Gale's term—Miracle Intervals—had a double meaning for fat people like me. It was a miracle that it worked and a miracle that it didn't kill me. Rest is so amazing!

> Gale's Miracle Intervals involved short intervals of high acceleration, followed by long recoveries at a slower pace. This was a fat-burning secret that changed my exercise regimen.

Better still, the science supported Gale's concept. In particular, she cited a research study that investigated the effects of short-term, high-intensity sprint-training on seventeen cyclists.

For the experiment, sprint-training workouts occurred twice per week for four weeks. The first workout included four thirty-second sprints followed by four minutes of active recovery. Two sprints were added to each training session. The total sprint work equaled twenty-eight minutes accumulated over the four weeks. The remainder of the training for the sprint group was endurance training. The result of the study was dramatic: "These data suggest that four weeks of high-intensity sprint training combined with endurance training in a trained cycling population increased motor unit activation, exercising plasma levels, and total work output with a relatively low volume of sprint exercise compared to endurance training alone."

The science showed that with a relatively low volume of sprint work, there was more muscle activation—that is, more muscles worked to contribute to the exercise load. Scientists also found that peak and mean (average) power outputs for the sprint cyclists improved, which translates to higher speeds. Sprint training improved performance compared to steady endurance training alone.

Results like this increased Gale's confidence in Miracle Intervals.

MIRACLE INTERVALS IMPROVE INSULIN SENSITIVITY

When Gale began using Miracle Intervals with me, I noticed two things right away: First, my overall speed was improving. And second, I didn't feel as hungry after my workouts. Further research revealed the reason. Short, high-intensity intervals improve insulin sensitivity. One study analyzed ten healthy men and compared the results of four all-out thirty-second sprints with continuous exercise at two levels—high intensity and low intensity. The researchers found that both exercise modes—short, high-intensity accelerations followed by a longer period at a slower pace—improved insulin sensitivity for forty-eight hours post-exercise. However, when they examined insulin sensitivity within thirty minutes of the end of the workouts, the thirty-second intervals improved insulin sensitivity better than the continuous exercise. The researchers concluded: "After a single exercise bout, four all-out thirty-second sprints acutely improve insulin sensitivity above continuous exercise."

Miracle Intervals were a *miraculous* revelation. But it gets better when combined with even more revelations about syncing workouts with the right diet strategy.

THE HIGH-OCTANE FOOD SECRET

Gale observed that many people think exercising hard for an hour can "burn off" that doughnut/greasy burger/ice cream sundae they've eaten. That idea, which is dead wrong, perhaps helps to explain why some top athletes end up with health and weight problems. For example, even endurance exercise experts, such as Dr. Tim Noakes, university professor and author of the book *The Lore of Running*, have come forward and revealed that they are having health problems that used to be reserved for an inactive population. Dr. Noakes has been diagnosed with diabetes.

How can people that exercise and eat healthfully be getting diabetes and coronary heart disease? While a few exercise experts with insulin problems and coronary heart disease might seem easy to brush off, multiple research papers have found troubling results. Two studies found that marathon racers were puzzlingly plagued with increased coronary heart disease problems. Another study found a high incidence of insulin resistance and coronary heart disease in nondiabetics.

Gale explained to me that some of the athletes she'd trained had faced similar struggles to mine. Like me, they'd questioned what was wrong with their exercise or nutrition program that was holding them back. They were following all of the conventional guidelines to a T. Why were the results so poor?

The answer might be in the types of food they were eating. Before we met, Gale had been experimenting with the effects of consuming higher percentages of fat and combining this change with tricks that endurance athletes have known for years. For example, it was proven years ago that doing a morning workout on an empty stomach promoted higher fat utilization than when people were fed before a workout. This was completely counter to conventional wisdom, which held that you needed to eat before a workout to keep your energy up.

But the most dramatic experimenting Gale was performing had to do with her fat intake. She told me that she'd observed a pattern among athletes and coaches in recent years. In particular, she'd noticed it in what she called the "ultrarunning" community. Granted, ultrarunners, who were capable of running up to one hundred miles on foot in fifteen to thirty hours, were an exceptional group—not like you and I! Most people wouldn't even want to do this, much less be able to. But their experience is instructive. These athletes were telling Gale that they were eating daily diets consisting of 70 percent fat.

A diet this high in fat seemed unreasonable. Insane. Unhealthy. But the anecdotal reports just kept rolling in to Gale, year after year. Not only were their daily diets high in fat, they were claiming to run events that take some fifteen to thirty hours on a mere 1,300 to 2,000 calories.

At first, this exercise intake seemed completely unbelievable to Gale. It's common knowledge in exercise science that the human body stores some 1,500 to 2,000 calories worth of glycogen (the stored form of glucose) in the muscles and liver. Glycogen is the easy to access and readily available fuel that the body uses for long exercise efforts. Also common knowledge is that a person exercising at high intensity can only do so for about ninety minutes before that readily accessible glycogen is depleted.

Glycogen depletion has been nicknamed "the bonk." Exercisers will do anything to avoid the bonk because it is so awful. Your mind wants to continue, but your body simply won't continue at the desired pace. Runners are reduced to a walk, and cyclists are forced to decrease average speed. Hikers, golfers, and skiers feel weak and lightheaded. Performance is severely, negatively affected. I know the bonk, and it isn't pretty. As I was losing weight with Dr. Lefkowitz, there were several times that I could feel it—on the golf course, during a race, or even during a long day at work. It isn't easy to fix once it happens. Once you're in it, you can't just eat your way out of it.

To avoid the bonk, endurance athletes are advised to consume 150 to 350 carbohydrate calories per hour in order to be capable of doing high-intensity exercise beyond ninety minutes. So when ultrarunners claimed to get by on so few calories—and more fat calories at that—it was just unbelievable. But Gale found that scientific research was catching up to the phenomenon. Science was now proving that athletes could burn more body fat and spare carbohydrates during exercise. The result is they need fewer supplemental calories during exercise.

MORE THAN JUST ANECDOTAL EVIDENCE

Gale had been following with interest an ongoing study on athletic performance and a high-fat diet conducted by Dr. Jeff Volek, a professor in the Department of Human Sciences at Ohio State University. His findings seemed to parallel her own experiences.

Dr. Volek's study compared two sets of evenly matched elite male distance runners. The first set of ten runners followed a traditional high-carbohydrate diet, with 60 percent of calories coming from carbohydrates, 25 percent from fat, and 15 percent from protein. The second set of runners followed a low-carbohydrate diet, with a mere 10 to 12 percent of calories coming from carbohydrates, a whopping 70 percent from fat, and around 20 percent from protein. The results showed that the fat-adapted athletes burned more fat at higher paces than the traditional carbohydrate diet group. For endurance athletes this means a significantly lower need for supplemental carbohydrates during training and racing, because more fat is being utilized as fuel.

This study was a game changer in Gale's thinking—evidence of a breakthrough in fitness and performance.

THE BOTTOM LINE: FAT BURNS, CARBOHYDRATE STORES

What does this evidence mean for ordinary exercisers? That fat, not carbs, is the high-octane fuel that makes you a Fat-Burning Machine.

Gale explained to me the details of the study in terms I could understand: Let's assume that our high-carbohydrate-runner is cruising along at a pace that burns up 500 calories per hour, so we can put the formula into different terms. Using the percentages from the study and translating back to calories, this high-carbohydrate-diet runner is burning around 200 calories per hour of carbohydrates and 300 calories of fat during exercise.

To keep it easy for comparison, say our runner has a friend who follows a fat-adapted diet, is the same body size, and can run the same pace as the high-carbohydrate-diet runner. This runner also burns 500 calories per hour, for the sake of simplicity. However, because this runner trained on a high-fat diet, she only used 10 percent carbohydrates and 90 percent fat to fuel the run.

Translating back to calories, the high-fat-diet runner is burning roughly 50 calories per hour of carbohydrates and 450 calories of fat.

In summary, our two theoretical athletes are exercising at a pace that burns 500 calories per hour. Our high-carbohydrate-diet runner is burning through carbohydrates at a rate of 200 calories per hour, and our fat-adapted-diet runner is only burning through 50 carbohydrate calories per hour. This is a huge difference.

The high-carb-diet athlete who is training for longer events will try to eat more—typically more carbohydrates—to make up for the lower level of fat burning. Often, athletes attempting to consume high amounts of carbohydrates per hour, particularly simple sugars, end up with stomach distress. This can lead to general discomfort or even vomiting.

Remember, we store only 1,300 to 2,000 calories of glycogen to fuel working muscles. However, fat stores are well in excess of 50,000 calories for most people. It is obvious that utilizing more fat to fuel exercise is beneficial for the endurance athlete.

> Gale's Burn Equation—Miracle Intervals + high-octane foods—addressed my metabolic syndrome and enhanced my fitness level. I was losing weight without being tired and hungry.

GALE DEBUNKS THE MYTH OF "ENERGY FOODS" FOR WORKOUTS

People who exercise often feel entitled to consume sugar and carbohydrates in the name of improved performance. Somehow, research studies on improving endurance performance got translated, misinterpreted, and mutilated to a terrible and deadly set of messages.

The wrong message: If you want to exercise better and improve performance for all exercise, you need to . . .

- Eat high-carbohydrate snacks or sports bars before all workouts.

- Drink a sugary sports drink during all exercise sessions, no matter the length or intensity.

- Consume a recovery drink that is high in carbohydrates and protein so you help your body repair from workouts—no matter the intensity or duration.

- Eat and drink high-sugar and high-carbohydrate sports products as snack foods and meals—even when no exercise is involved.

All of these statements are absolutely false. By continuing these practices, you are doing nothing but training your body to efficiently store fat, even if you exercise. Worse yet, you are harming your health.

Energy drinks have evolved in diverse directions from the original sports drinks that were made to help athletes recover from physical exertion. These beverages claim to work by altering blood sugar levels with the purpose of increasing endurance, energy, and performance. Despite the claims, scientific evidence refutes these assertions. Instead, energy drinks may interfere with normal body mechanisms to signal that you are tired. They may also carry more serious health consequences.

The human body has an effective means for managing blood sugar, primarily through the action of two hormones, insulin and glucagon. When blood sugar levels rise after eating or through other stimuli, the pancreas releases insulin to restore blood glucose to normal levels. During activity, the pancreas releases glucagon that, in turn, stimulates the metabolism of stored sugars to increase blood sugar to meet the body's need for energy.

Energy drinks contain ingredients that may alter blood sugar levels. Some beverages contain added sugars that can manipulate sugar levels and bypass the normal feedback system. Others may contain caffeine or other stimulants. These substances fool the body into thinking it's in a fight-or-flight type of situation. In response to this, the body releases epinephrine or adrenaline. Blood sugar levels may rise to ensure adequate energy availability. In a sensitive individual, this effect can lead to hyperglycemia or abnormally high blood sugar.

> I didn't have to eat lots of carbs to get more energy for exercise. No more loading up on pasta or sugar-laden drinks for workouts. Burning fat not carbs was the high-octane secret.

So don't be so fast to grab an energy bar or slug down an energy drink—before, during, or after exercise—especially if the workout duration is an hour or so. Rather than gaining more energy for performance, you might be sabotaging your entire effort.

THE BURN EQUATION WORKS

Gale's Burn Equation—Miracle Intervals plus high-octane foods—not only addressed my metabolic syndrome; it also enhanced my entire fitness program. The Fat-Burning Machine Diet and workout program in this book shows you how to do it.

This isn't just about becoming an athlete. It's about living well. The primary reason for exercise is to enable you to maintain a high quality of life for as long as possible. It's about being mobile, doing your daily errands, doing the things you enjoy at the drop of a hat. It's about not missing out on family activities because you have trouble walking more than a block. It's about being strong, not feeble.

In the workout plans in Part Two of this book, you will find specific exercise intensity instructions designed to improve fitness and teach your body how to be a Fat-Burning Machine. But know that exercise alone is not enough for the results you're seeking. Your daily nutrition has a significant effect on how your body responds to exercise. Though this program is likely higher in fat than what you've seen in past exercise book recommendations, you can relax knowing it is *not* a 70 percent fat diet.

When you combine daily dietary food habits to promote fat burning, along with nutrition practices during exercise that also promote fat burning, you have a winning combination.

Training with Gale was truly a magical process for me; she opened up a world of fitness that I knew existed but never believed I could be a part of. One of the reasons that I loved triathlons was the culture. People who run triathlons are serious. They have a common bond of training—hours in the pool, miles on the bike, and exhausting runs in sweltering heat. They share many life experiences. They struggle with balancing their work, life, and training. And they know how to perform in the races. With Gale's help, I wanted to go through the looking glass; I wanted to learn their secrets; I wanted to unlock my athletic potential and be able to perform in these races. Finishing the triathlons was no longer enough. I was always the fat kid who couldn't break an eight-minute mile or the swimmer who struggled to do the one-hundred-yard freestyle in under a minute.

Gale and I have developed a customized nutrition plan that synced to my fitness in an innovative way; I could now burn the energy that I had stored as fat rather than feeling like I had to eat more.

We blazed our own trail using the best athletic science and adapted it for people like me who store fat rather than burn it. We planned our nutrition as carefully as we planned our fitness. In this book, you'll find instructions for short workouts with speed accelerations to get the Fat-Burning Machine running and keep it running all day; longer workouts in the morning at a pace that uses only stored glycogen; and weight training to build lower-body strength and to shape the body.

The results were stunning. My 10K times dropped in each race I ran. I ran personal records in my half marathons. My early season Olympic distance triathlon in Naples was a personal record for me. I completed the Half Ironmans in Orlando, Syracuse, and Maine. The length and speeds of my bike rides increased even in twenty-degree temperatures. I was setting the pace for my lane in the pool.

And as I increased my training and distances, my weight was steadily dropping again. My body was changing. Finally. My clothes were starting to become loose. My belt tightened. My shirts became baggy. People who I hadn't seen for awhile said that I looked "fit." I was experiencing other benefits as well. As I described earlier, my skin looked ten years younger, I slept better, I felt much more energy, and some of the health problems—acid reflux, joint pain—that had plagued me for years simply disappeared. I realized that I was, at last, a Fat-Burning Machine. I was curious to know if my experience could be duplicated by others. Gale and I put together a test group of people to try the Fat-Burning Diet program, including people representing a variety of ages and physical conditions. We were thrilled when the members of our test group constantly achieved great results. That's why we decided to write this book to reach a wider audience with a program that works. Now it's your turn!

FOUR

COMPLETE YOUR FITNESS BUCKET LIST

Everyone Deserves to Succeed

People were always telling me that what I wanted from life wasn't possible. But once I ignored the doubters, I found my path. I knew I couldn't possibly be the only active, athletic guy who gained weight. And I wasn't going to let it stay that way. I didn't give up, and I finally found the method that worked. So my message to you is: *You can do it—even if you've never succeeded before.* So, let's talk about you. Can you relate to my fat-storing experience? Are you frustrated and looking for answers?

Everyone has a fitness bucket list. Maybe it's halting the slide into an extra pound every year; maybe it's running a marathon; maybe it's having the energy to move confidently through a day; maybe it's all of the above. It's a funny thing about bucket lists. They represent our hopes and dreams, right? But we also tend to shove them on a shelf, because hoping and dreaming don't seem to work so well. Bucket lists always seem beyond our reach.

And motivation can be hard to maintain when things aren't working. It might not surprise you to know that research shows most people who try diets end up going back to their normal routine in less than three weeks, and the process of gaining weight starts again—a pound at a time, a quarter inch by a quarter inch, until it's back. And when people gain it back, they usually gain a little more weight than when they started. They get a little bigger and even more frustrated. That's the cycle.

If that's happened to you, you've probably felt like a giant failure. What you probably didn't realize is that's the *real plan* of all of the diets you tried. In fact, there is a whole industry that depends on it. They're based on the premise that people have to gain a little extra weight back in order to become even hungrier for a solution. And the beat goes on. Believe me, they don't mind if you feel like a failure. It is time to share the secrets no one in the diet industry wants you to know. It is time to stop playing their game.

Remember, I was the guy with shelves full of books who had tried them all. It was an agonizing process and even worse because I never succeeded. I feel that people shouldn't have to pay thousands of dollars to nutritionists to get the same old meal plans that are not sustainable. I mean, really? Do you have to buy a book or hire a nutritionist to tell you to eat fewer carbs, exercise more, and drink plenty of water? It's an insult to your intelligence.

It's time to get rid of the fat-shaming culture. If you're like me, one of the worst things about putting on the pounds is the realization that other people are judging you. Nobody thinks you can be active and overweight. *Nobody.* When I was training for the New York City Marathon and putting on ten pounds, I know people would say, "Who gains ten pounds running a marathon?" I tried to rationalize it by saying the extra weight must be muscle. Yeah, right. If I really looked inside, I would have said that I *did* feel shame. But why? That's when I really knew that it wasn't me, it was something else—a secret I had to know.

It's also time to let go of the notion that if you're overweight you're messed up psychologically. You've heard and maybe used the descriptions: "I'm an emotional eater." "I can't control my cravings." "I don't have the discipline." "I guess I'm a quitter." You beat yourself up. Again, these are all just rationalizations that have to stop.

The first time I went to see Dr. Lefkowitz and she told me about metabolic syndrome, it was like having a boulder lifted off my stomach. It wasn't emotional; it was physical. What a revelation! Suddenly my history of struggling with weight loss made sense to me. I could stop blaming myself—or my genes—and get to work. Dr. Lefkowitz, and then Gale, opened my eyes to a whole new way to approaching my weight. It was totally different than anything I'd ever tried before. And ultimately, the plan, which is offered in this book, was a path to a lifestyle change that felt good and worked.

> Finally, I'm a Fat-Burning Machine and I'm not afraid of "falling off" the wagon. There is no wagon. No fad. No extreme protocol. Just a way of life that combines science and practical strategies.

Finally, I'm a Fat-Burning Machine and I'm not afraid of "falling off" the wagon. There is no wagon. No fad. No extreme protocol. Just a way of life that combines science and practical strategies. A method to keep the fat off for good. Learning the secrets gave me power over my weight and fitness for the first time in my life. I can't wait to pass along those secrets to you. Just by opening this book, you are on your way to becoming a Fat-Burning Machine.

ARE YOU READY?

So let's get to work. Ask yourself:

- Have you been gaining a pound or so a year, for the past few years?

- Do you crave sugar and snacks and worry that you can't control your cravings?

- Is your waistline slowly increasing? Bit by bit, year by year? Do you have a muffin top?

- Do you love being active, but find that hours spent at the gym or on the trail or at the tennis court don't stop the pounds from piling on? (Worse still, do you find that heavier exercise leads to *more* weight gain?)

- Do you feel that the more you exercise, the hungrier you are and the more you eat?

- Does exercise make you feel tired and weak?

- Do your blood tests or measurements show that you have any or many of the signs of metabolic syndrome: large waist circumference, high LDL cholesterol, low HDL cholesterol, high blood pressure, high triglycerides, high glucose? (Remember, even if you have one or two your body might be conditioned to be a fat-storing machine.)

- Are you tired of failing?

- Do you look on enviously as others seem to effortlessly achieve the things that are on your bucket list?

If you answered yes to these questions, this book is for you and you're ready to start your transformation from a fat-storing machine to a Fat-Burning Machine.

If you're like me, you have to combat many barriers to achieving your bucket list, including old habits that are preventing you from being a Fat-Burning Machine. And contrary to popular belief, those habits probably aren't laziness or gorging on sweets and fatty foods. I thought I ate pretty healthfully. I wasn't a fast-food addict. Obviously, I wasn't a couch potato. I learned that my "bad" habits were more nuanced—things I did because I thought they would help me, but they actually only made my condition worse. And once I learned the secrets of how to eat and exercise in a way that was calibrated for fat burning, my life changed.

OUR PROMISE

Whether you are running triathlons like me, taking walks, playing tennis on the weekends, or riding your bike, Gale and I will keep your Fat-Burning Machine running strong so that you can stay fit and perform for the rest of your life.

I know it can feel a little scary when you're first starting in a new direction. You'll have to learn new things and let go of old ideas and habits. Some of your most closely held beliefs about diet and fitness will get smashed. I've been there, so I understand those feelings. But now, I believe we've cracked the formula. For the first time, we're offering a way for you to be a Fat-Burning Machine—and stay that way. Most importantly, you will finally understand your body and what makes it perform better. You will engineer your body to burn fat rather than store it. As your life changes, you'll find that the items on your bucket list aren't so impossible after all.

It's an irresistible possibility, and as you read the secrets Gale and I will share with you, you'll see that you can achieve that goal. Nothing would make me happier. Unlike most diet and fitness programs, I don't want you coming back for more and more and more. I want you to live your life.

So take your bucket list off the shelf, and let's get going.

FIVE

LET'S HIT RESET

These Ten Myths Are Sabotaging Your Success

It's time to hit the reset button, and that starts with purging your mind of a few misconceptions. We all have them. When I started my journey to become a Fat-Burning Machine, I realized that over a lifetime I had adopted some "truths" about food, exercise, and dieting that I believed absolutely. I have no idea of their origin or where I picked up the information, but after a lifetime of carrying them around in my head, they had become elevated to the level of irrefutable fact. But guess what? They were completely false.

As I look back, it surprises me that I could be so off. Nearly every notion that I had was wrong. And yet, each of them was rooted in some sort of fact. I didn't make it up, but my interpretation or application was wrong.

Here are the top ten myths that are sabotaging your success.

1. DIETS WORK. I'M THE PROBLEM.

On most diets I tried, I initially lost some weight, but none of them worked on a long-term basis. I always thought it was my fault that I was overweight. I just couldn't control my eating. The formula was straightforward: I needed to go on a diet (any diet) and stick with it.

Then my weight problem would be solved. In my mind, the diets were all good. I was the bad one. I was the problem, not the diet. I had no willpower.

As I look back, there was no way that those diets were going to work beyond the start. I was a fat-storing machine. It wasn't willpower. It was my body makeup. My body chemistry was set up in such a way that each diet was just making me fatter by making me more insulin resistant. If I was losing weight, it was because I was eating less in the beginning. But in reality, many of these diets were subversively teaching my body to optimize fat storing, rather than fat burning. Sure, I lost weight initially, but as soon as I went back to my normal eating, I ended up heavier than when I began.

THE RESET: I needed to treat the underlying syndrome, not just the isolated symptoms. Sure, I could have gone one by one, addressing my high cholesterol, my high blood sugar, my ever-expanding waist—but they were part of a package. The underlying dynamics that caused my symptoms had to be understood and addressed head-on, with changes to my nutrition and fitness that could be sustained.

---

2. A GOOD WORKOUT IS A SWEAT STORM.

I like being active and don't mind sweating, but I thought that in order to lose weight I would have to thoroughly soak my T-shirt and have sweat pouring down my face. I had this image that fitness for people like me was a boot camp drill sergeant screaming at me, shaming me and making me feel bad about myself, making me huff and puff. I felt inadequate enough about being overweight; did I really need some guy with 7 percent body fat telling me I could do better? Unfortunately, this idea has gained purchase in the culture, thanks to programs like *The Biggest Loser*. That's the real shame.

But the idea has been around for a long time. Many years go, during a summer internship in New York, my boss heard that I was bothered by the weight I'd gained in college and how out of shape

I was. He volunteered to be my trainer. I was young, so this didn't seem weird to me at the time. I thought of it as a good way to spend more time with the boss, so I agreed. He took me to his fancy gym, and as soon as we got there, he put me on the scale. I was mortified to see what I weighed, and embarrassed that he knew as well. He spent the next few weeks making me run on the treadmill until I couldn't stop sweating. It was truly gross. Afterward, he would take me to Papaya King, the local juice place in New York, and buy me a "healthy" banana shake to recover. I would burn off 300 calories at the gym and drink 500 calories as my recovery drink. Not good, but at the time I had no idea the sabotage that was happening. Needless to say, I gained weight that summer. My boss—maybe to save face—assured me it was muscle. I know better now.

Exercise and fitness were intimidating and off-putting to me. I never performed well. The idea of being tortured for even fifteen minutes, let alone half an hour, was just so unappealing. Constant agony, out of breath, falling behind everyone, drenched. Why would I do that?

THE RESET: I never liked the gym, and I still don't. Exercise and being fit are all about personal choices. I found that I liked to exercise outdoors with goals in mind, and that's why I started entering races. I liked to do a variety of sports, so sometimes I swam, sometimes I ran, other times I would bike and in the winters even ski. During one summer, I decided to keep fit by carrying my golf bag on my shoulder and walking eighteen holes.

> Exercise and being fit are all about personal choices.

The point is that fitness worked best for me when it fit into my lifestyle. Not the other way around. What did I like to do? What gave me pleasure? What was I good at? I had to enjoy fitness to keep at it. So simple, yet so true.

The conventional wisdom of long, slow workouts (and a lot of them) being the best way to manage weight loss was going to take a lot of time and bore me to death. The worst part is that it would have little to no positive impact. Burning fat actually requires mixing it up and igniting your body's fat-burner.

I learned that short, high-intensity exercise not only utilizes fat for fuel, it also influences insulin reaction and helps build the networks of capillaries that will later assist in making your body a Fat-Burning Machine. Longer duration and less intense exercise utilizes a greater percentage of fat for fuel within a certain intensity range. The point is that both have a role. Just sweating isn't the answer.

---

3. YOU HAVE TO BE HUNGRY TO LOSE WEIGHT.

I always equated weight loss with hunger pains. If my stomach was roaring and my mind was consumed with cravings for the food I couldn't have, I was doing well. If I was dreaming of the next time I would eat, I was doing well. I was conditioned to believe that you couldn't lose weight unless you could feel the emptiness in your stomach. Feeling full was a recipe for guilt. It probably meant you were cheating.

I would brag to people about the meals I was skipping. Being hungry was a badge of honor that I proudly wore on my chest. I loved to skip breakfast or "work through lunch." But I could always feel it, and by the time I got to the next meal, I was ravenous. Like a killer whale going through a school of fish, I would eat everything I could as fast as I could. Denying myself food just set me up to overeat—and usually with the wrong foods. When you're starving, you don't take the time to make a nice salad!

THE RESET: Now I realize that I should feel satisfied by the food I eat, and if I am not, I should eat something more. Being hungry is exactly the wrong feeling for sustainable weight loss and a healthy lifestyle. It is *what* I eat that is key. I could not eat something that would trigger my insulin and make me even hungrier.

I need complex carbohydrates loaded with vitamins, minerals, and

5. FRUIT IS NATURAL, SO IT MUST BE GOOD FOR YOU.

While I never really liked vegetables until recently, I have always loved fruit. All types of fruit—apples, oranges, grapes, watermelon, cantaloupe, bananas, strawberries. In the summer, my favorite meal was a huge fruit salad. I would buy whole watermelons, chop them up, and just eat them throughout the day.

How bad could it be for me? Even if it is sweet, the sugar in fruit is natural, not processed. God-given from the tree or the vine, right? I thought I should be able to eat it in unlimited quantities. After a workout, I would love to have a juicy red apple or two (or three). It would taste so good, quench my thirst, and help me recover. When I was training, I was told to eat bananas to prevent cramping and to facilitate recovery. Little did I know that bananas were loaded with sugar and were sabotaging the impact of my workouts and making me hungrier.

THE RESET: The more fruit I ate, the hungrier it made me. The sugar levels in fruit were triggering my fat-storing machine. While some fruits have less sugar than others, eating fruit made me want more fruit. I'm not saying that you have to eliminate fruit. It has its place. But it's not the abundant cornucopia we think it is. (See the list of high-sugar, medium-sugar, and low-sugar fruits on page 81.)

---

6. WEIGHT LIFTING WILL MAKE YOU BULKY AND HEAVY

I have naturally broad shoulders and a barrel chest. When I gain weight, one of the first places I see it is in my chest. Fear of bulking up made me very reluctant to try any sort of weight lifting.

Weight lifting also looked very hard. All of those weights! It was intimidating, to say the least. I cringed listening to the grunting and groaning that people made when they were lifting. I hated the slamming noise that the weights made. It seemed very scary for me.

There was no way I would be able to do this myself. I would need a trainer to show me the ins and outs, and I could only picture an image of the trainer barking at me.

phytochemicals, combined with fat and protein to engage my F
Burning Machine. My morning had to begin with a great breakfast
would sabotage the rest of the day. I started to plan fat-burning snac
to keep my energy high, hunger low, and eliminate fat storing.

Eating frequent small meals and snacks throughout the day
much better for me than eating fewer larger meals. Frequent mea
keep my hormones at a stable level and my Fat-Burning Machine ru
ning.

When blood sugar is stabilized, the body releases insulin to utili
food as fuel, rather than to store it as fat. Exercise combined with th
wrong food choices causes hunger, stunts insulin release, and encou
ages fat storage.

4. HEALTHY FOOD ISN'T YUMMY.

Looking back, I must have completely made this one up based on th
conventional wisdom perpetuated by the food industry. It was merel
a rationalization of why I ate some foods and didn't eat others. And
yet, so many people believe the same thing. I know that I am not alone.

It had nothing to do with the taste or texture of food; it had to
do with my palate and what I was used to eating. Truthfully, what
is more disgusting than potatoes, fried in oil with salt? But I loved
them. Sometimes, I would order a club sandwich and double fries. I
couldn't get enough, and the more I ate, the more I wanted.

I had to have rice or pasta with every meal that I ate. It seemed
like it was balancing everything out. I was sabotaging myself every
night. Who knew?

THE RESET: It took some time to change the food I liked. I literally had
to train my palate to like fresh vegetables. How? By eating them and
preparing them in ways that were enjoyable. At first, I only liked carrots.
To the point that I turned orange I ate so many. Gradually I became more
adventurous and moved on to broccoli, cauliflower, even the dreaded
Brussels sprouts. Now I like them.

Having said that, when I did go to the gym, I did enjoy the machines—the crunch one that you did for your abs, the shoulder press with cool grips and bars, and the hydraulic lift machine that helped me do a pull-up (couldn't remember the last time that I did one of those before I was a Fat-Burning Machine). The problem was, I just couldn't really figure out how it fit into my life and therefore was able to dismiss it.

THE RESET: Once I started lifting weights, beginning with small hand weights, I noticed that instead of making me bigger, adding weights to my workout made me stronger and more toned. I was able to reshape my body with weights. Strength training builds muscle and improves quality of life. I also found out that muscle is more metabolically active than fat. Fat-Burning Machines run more efficiently with strong muscles, particularly a strong lower body. I never really liked doing lunges and squats, but they work long after my workout is finished—even when I'm sleeping!

The key challenge was how to fold strength training into an aerobic program—or how to fold an aerobic program into strength training. I needed to combine the two. Doing too much of one or the other wouldn't work.

I found that strength training was of equal importance to aerobic training. Aerobic training works to improve the cardiovascular (heart, blood vessels) and the pulmonary (lungs) systems. Strength training improves muscular strength, balance, and coordination. Strength training is important to bone density, so that I don't become feeble and brittle.

---

7. BITES, LICKS, AND TASTES DON'T COUNT.

I love to have just a bite or a lick of something. Some of the things that I ate were worthy of a taste—a delicious piece of chocolate cake with vanilla ice cream, hot bread fresh out of the oven, guacamole with crisp, salty nacho chips.

Other less worthy things came straight off my kids' plates—

macaroni and cheese, cold pizza, or baked ziti that they left after it had seen better days. It didn't really matter if the food was good or not. I would eat indiscriminately. I was of the mind-set that it was easier to eat it off their plate than throw it away. I justified it by saying it was "just a taste."

I thought, what was the big deal? Those bites, licks, and tastes were too small to make a difference or have impact. After all, I wasn't eating the whole plate—I was just nibbling or sampling. There is a big difference. Notably, I never wanted to have a taste of healthy foods like zucchini or plain Greek yogurt. My tastes always involved something sweet or high in carbohydrates. Again, it came back to my palate and brain being impulsive for those types of foods.

I see this at the supermarket, when they put out food for people to taste: a piece of pound cake, a cracker with a cheese spread, a taste of pasta, or tiny sausages with mustard. The stores aren't stupid—they know what they are doing. They are spiking your insulin to make you hungry so you will buy more.

THE RESET: No matter how harmless my bites, licks, and tastes seemed at the time, they weren't worth it. They were never satisfying. I always wanted more, and they destabilized my hormones. They sabotaged all of my good work. No matter how balanced I had eaten the rest of the day, it could all be undone by one bite (that was never really one bite anyway).

---

8. A HEALTHY DIET MEANS AVOIDING FAT.

I totally bought into the idea that I had to eliminate all fat from my diet. I started buying nonfat foods. I stopped eating cheese. I found the fat-free versions of mayonnaise, yogurt, and cottage cheese. If it said "fat-free," I was in. Even avocados were to be avoided. For my salads, only balsamic vinegar would do. As a result, I was starving all the time, particularly if I was exercising more.

Also, most of the processed food that is supposedly low in fat is high in carbohydrates. Just the opposite of what I was trying to do.

THE RESET: Fat around your gut is bad, but fat in food is not necessarily the enemy. I found that I had to keep the levels of fat up in my diet to feel full and satisfied. Fat provides energy and improves your health markers. It is fat in combination with highly refined carbohydrates or plain sugar that turns off your Fat-Burning Machine.

> Fat around your gut is bad, but fat in food is not necessarily the enemy.

It is more beneficial to blend the diet based on activity and exercise. This blend may well change from meal to meal, depending on your activity. For example, begin with a diet that is 35 percent fat, 35 percent protein, and 30 percent carbohydrate. As your activity level increases, you may find you need to add more carbohydrates and decrease fat or protein.

---

9. IT IS BETTER TO CHEAT IN THE MORNING SO YOU CAN BURN IT OFF.

No one is perfect. I certainly wasn't. Everyone strays. For me, bagels with cream cheese were a huge temptation. Or ice cream. I had heard somewhere if I was going to go off my plan, I should do it in the morning so I could spend the rest of the day "working" it off.

But it never seemed to go that way. Once I cheated in the morning, my metabolic syndrome kicked in and I was hungrier all day—especially craving rich carbs and fat. And, psychologically, cheating early set me up with a rationalization to cheat for the rest of the day. I would think, well, I had a bagel with cream cheese for breakfast, how bad can this cheeseburger be at lunch or maybe just a small bowl of this delicious spaghetti Bolognese at dinner?

I could never stop cheating once I started. I would be hungry all day long, with huge cravings for food that could only be satisfied by carbs. It was so weird. On most days, I wasn't even tempted, but once I started I couldn't stop. I wondered if this is how alcoholics felt. Was I so addicted and susceptible to sugar and carbs that they could have this impact on me?

And yet, the next day I would wake up and it would be back to normal. This insatiable appetite for carbs never carried over from day to day.

THE RESET: So, I had it completely wrong. If I was going to cheat, breakfast or lunch was exactly the wrong time because of the domino effect it would have on the rest of my day. It didn't matter if I could burn off my calories. I couldn't get my insulin stabilized, no matter how much exercise I did. The truth is that you can't overcome a bad diet through exercise alone. Exercise can help make your body more fit, but it will not promote weight loss.

If I was going to treat myself to ice cream or pasta, it was much better to do it at dinner. The benefit was that I had less time to compound the problem I was creating for myself, and the next day I could be careful.

---

10. A DIET IS MISERY—ALWAYS.

I always believed that when you are on a diet you have to suffer. You know the expression—"no pain, no gain." If you actually like the food that you are eating on your diet, you will eat too much of it and it won't work. I think this idea goes back to my past when I tended to binge on food. Once I started with a bag of potato chips, I wouldn't stop until it was done. If I ordered Chinese takeout, I had a bad habit of finishing it all, no matter when I became full.

So my logic was that an effective diet involved foods that I didn't actually want to eat. I figured if I didn't like something, I wouldn't be tempted to binge on it.

But why did I have to suffer? Was it possible to actually enjoy the new foods I was eating so I wouldn't miss the old foods so much? I didn't want to live my whole life hating what was on my plate.

THE RESET: You have to like the food that you are eating if you want to have a sustainable lifestyle. Meals are an essential social part of our lives. You don't want to be the one at the dinner party miserably nibbling on a lettuce leaf. If you don't like the food you are eating, you are depriving yourself of one of the great joys of life. You will also not be able to stay on the plan.

Instead of denying yourself, find foods that you like on the plan. When I started eating to become a Fat-Burning Machine, I found so many new foods that I loved and now look forward to—my creative egg white omelets in the morning, the inventive salads with chicken that I have for lunch, and dinners that use fish and vegetables and other fresh ingredients, blending flavors and textures in a mouthwatering way. I love the excitement of going to different restaurants and discovering amazing dishes that I never would have ordered before. It forces me to be more aware of the benefits and the consequences of different meals. And the payoff is that I can love what I'm eating without guilt or fear of sliding back.

There are probably other misconceptions lurking out there. Maybe you have some of your own. You can recognize them by their rigid absoluteness and by the fact that they don't stand the test of real life experience. Remember, your goal is to live your life, not to put on a straitjacket. I think you'll find that once you hit reset on your old notions, you'll feel an exhilarating freedom—and also relief. There's nothing worse than following a path that you know from past experience doesn't lead to your goal. This time when you start, you'll be armed with science and truth to get you where you want to go.

Now, let's get started.

PART TWO

THE FAT-BURNING MACHINE PROGRAM

—

SIX

GETTING STARTED

Understand the Markers that Matter

For the first forty-two years of my life, I practiced various forms of avoidance and petty deception to escape the reality of my condition. The regular measures of my health and weight were sources of fear and disappointment. I thought the best way to keep track of my weight was to weigh myself on my bathroom scale, but it was something of a denial game. When I was feeling particularly fit, I would weigh myself more frequently. When I felt a little puffy, I would weigh myself less often. My rationale was that I couldn't officially be heavier if I didn't weigh myself. I could only gain weight if I actually *knew* what I weighed. So for many months I would go without weighing myself.

Like most people with weight issues, I had different clothes for my various sizes. There were my skinny clothes, my fat clothes, and some clothes that were in between. It actually made me very nervous getting dressed sometimes because I just didn't know if what I wanted to wear would actually fit. When things fit, I felt happy and good about myself; when they didn't, I felt disappointed and bummed out.

Of course, each year I went to my doctor for my annual checkup. I dreaded that appointment. The visit always started with a nurse weighing me on the "official" scale. I anxiously watched as she slowly moved the weights to the right. It was torture as she looked at the scale, looked back at my medical chart, and then adjusted the weight. Why did I always weigh more at the doctor's office than I did at home? Why did the nurse always have that look of judgment on her face like, "Uh-oh, Mike's weight is up again . . ."

After the weigh-in, the nurse started drawing blood from my left arm, which went into different colored bottles. She'd praise me for my great veins and how easy they were to find—which always made me feel proud. So much blood. What could they possibly be doing with so many separate vials?

My doctor would come in and tell me that I had gained a few pounds and I should consider watching what I ate (more veggies, less pasta), and she would suggest that I start exercising more regularly. A couple of weeks later, I'd get a letter from the doctor's office with the results of my blood work: just a bunch of numbers that made no sense to me. I never really cared or paid that much attention. The doctor's visit was something to be endured, the results something to ignore and deny.

It all kind of seemed like nothing interesting, nothing insightful. My weight was going up a pound or two a year, my blood numbers moving in the wrong direction, but nothing to really worry about. It didn't seem as if I could *do* anything with the information.

Then, a couple of years ago, before I decided to become a Fat-Burning Machine, my doctor actually called my home and wanted to speak to me. That was weird. What did she find? She said that my cholesterol numbers were high and she wanted to start me on a medication to reduce them. She explained that over the years, my bad cholesterol had been moving up and my good cholesterol moving down. After giving me a lecture about changing my diet (for the tenth straight year), she prescribed a drug to help with my cholesterol.

Suddenly, it wasn't the same old annual checkup. Was that it? The slippery slope was starting. Now I was going to be taking daily pills for the rest of my life? It certainly was a moment to stop and reflect. I took the pills for about a week and I had a bad reaction. They made me hot and itchy. They weren't for me. Something was going to have to change. It was a wake-up call.

As I looked at my health profile, I realized that the first thing to change was that I had to stop being so passive. Notice that all of the ways I was measuring my fitness were like out-of-body experiences. Someone (or something) was doing it to me. I was just standing there waiting for results, and half the time I closed my eyes and ears so I wouldn't have to acknowledge the truth. I had to take matters into my own hands. This was a big decision.

Embarking on a fitness program is not something that gets done to you. It's something you do for yourself. You have to put yourself in the driver's seat and decide to be a fully present participant. So before you get started, here are a few ideas.

EVALUATE YOUR MARKERS

As a career researcher, I believe in a simple concept: *Actions have consequences.* If you take a certain action, you can expect a certain result. I believe in predictable outcomes and measurable results. Outcomes are predictable because they are based on known facts, not random events. When you measure an outcome, it is called a result. Results should be measured to determine how closely they align with the prediction. If there is a difference, it should be explainable.

I apply this principle to virtually everything I do in my professional and personal life. I predict and I measure—it is what I do. As a political pollster, I develop campaigns and predict elections for my candidates based on polls. As an athlete, I train for triathlons and then I compete to see how I perform. I am much more surprised when things don't go the way I expect than when they do.

But this approach never worked with my weight. No matter what outcome I desired, I could never achieve the result I wanted. I mean, sure, from time to time I lost some weight, but it was always fleeting, and in the long run, I ended up heavier than when I started.

A big reason was that my inputs were wrong. I was expecting

predictable results without evaluating the right markers. As I began to understand the markers of metabolic syndrome, I realized that there were other factors that were important to predicting my weight.

- Increasingly high cholesterol

- A growing waist

- High blood sugar levels

These together suggested that my body was processing food differently than other people. I had a metabolism issue.

Losing weight was an outcome that was down the road. I had more immediate factors that I would have to address before I could truly impact my weight.

MAKE A SCHEDULE OF THE KEY MEASURES

As a practical matter, I knew that I couldn't measure everything, so I decided to establish three PPIs (Personal Performance Indicators) that I would measure on a regular basis:

1. My blood work (every six months)

2. My measurements (monthly)

3. My weight (weekly)

DO CALORIES COUNT?

There's one thing I never measure—calories. Let me explain.

As a political pollster, I love counting how many supporters we have and calculating how many more we need to win the election.

As a triathlete, I love counting how many miles I have completed in the race and figuring out how many more I have to go to finish.

As a golfer, I love counting how many strokes it took me to complete a round.

But as a Fat-Burning Machine, I have never liked to count calories. Unlike the other metrics in my world, calories are too imprecise. They are simply too hard, too unreliable, and too subjective to be a reliable measure.

Look, I know that if you eat fewer calories you will lose weight. It is a fact. And I do think it is really cool that many restaurants post calories on menus; people should be aware of the relative caloric count of one choice vs. another. But counting calories with any precision is only good in theory. It is virtually impossible to do in reality. Why? Because portion sizes vary and it is impossible to know each ingredient. And even if I could measure calories precisely, why would I want to? Think about how often I eat; why would I want to log each calorie? What an inconvenience. I needed to get beyond calories and to healthy choices. The calories would take care of themselves.

For me, calories become a source of rationalization for bad behavior and false hope. All calories are not created equal, and some have more negative impact than others. How many times have I justified eating or drinking something because it was "low-calorie" even though it had other negative consequences? A great example is diet soda. Sure, it has no calories, but what about the impact of the sweeteners mimicking sugar, the chemicals in my system? Would I still drink it if it were high in calories?

On the flip side, once I make the decision to eat something that is high in calories, do I really care if it is 500, 600, or 700 calories? How many calories does a slice of pizza have? Who cares? I am going off the plan. Might as well enjoy it.

As I said before, all calories are not equal. A piece of white meat chicken has the same calories as a Snickers bar. The white meat chicken has fifty-three grams of protein and no carbohydrates. The Snickers bar is thirty-three grams of carbohydrates and only four grams of protein. The choice is clear.

I only use calories on a relative basis. The same way I do for carbs. If some foods have more carbs than others, I choose the lower carb food. If some foods have more calories than others, it is a good idea to eat the lower calorie food.

As we all know, PPIs have to be simple to be effective. It takes less than ten minutes to establish your Fat-Burning Machine benchmarks from which you will set your goal and measure your progress for a lifetime. For most people, these are the same tests that get done at your annual checkup. But this time you're armed with an understanding of how to use them.

THE BLOOD WORK BENCHMARKS—EVERY SIX MONTHS

I never really understood the importance of blood work. I usually ignored the numbers on the page because they were confusing and I didn't know what they meant. Staring at those pages of numbers was like being asked to take an advanced chemistry exam. And even if I understood the numbers, what the hell was I going to do with them? But now I was going to have to start learning what to look for and why those numbers were important. Once I started doing that, I realized that my blood test was actually a crucial road map to my condition and a way to measure changes as I progressed.

Here's a simple checklist of the numbers you should look for in your blood test results.

- **Total cholesterol**—High cholesterol (over 200 mg/dL) is known as hypercholesterolemia and is a major risk factor for heart attack and stroke.

- **HDL**—High-density lipoproteins, considered the "good" cholesterol, are part of the total cholesterol number. Doctors want HDL to be greater than 60 mg/dL. Increasing your HDL number is associated with decreasing atherosclerosis or the narrowing and hardening of the arteries.

- **LDL**—Low-density lipoproteins, considered the "bad" cholesterol, are also part of the total cholesterol number. LDL collects on the walls of your blood vessels and causes atherosclerosis along with eventually causing complete blockages. Obviously not a good thing. Doctors want LDL to be less than 100 mg/dL.

- **Total Cholesterol/HDL**—Doctors like this ratio to be less than 3.5, ideally. When you get to 4.5 to 5.0, it is considered a health risk.

- **Triglycerides**—These, in addition to cholesterol, are a type of lipid or fat found in your blood. When you eat and the calories aren't used right away, the body converts these to triglycerides that are stored in your fat cells. Hormones can later release these lipids for energy between meals. The ideal is for triglycerides to measure less than 150 mg/dL. Borderline trouble is between 150 and 199 mg/dL. High triglyceride levels are associated with increased risk of heart disease.

- **Fasting glucose**—Doctors like this number to be between 60 and 99 mg/dL. If values are between 100 and 125 mg/dL, it is considered prediabetic.

A WORD ABOUT HORMONES

Two hormones are involved in the process of fat storing vs. fat burning. When I first heard about the role of hormones, I immediately thought back to sex-ed with Dr. Susan Humphrey at the Latin School in Chicago. But these were different hormones—the endocrine hormones that affected my weight. These hormones are chemical messengers that create fast-acting chemical controls for bodies, and I had to pay attention to them if I was going to succeed.

The two major endocrine hormones are insulin and cortisol. Insulin, as we discussed earlier, is the hormone made by the pancreas that helps the body use sugar (glucose) for energy. Insulin resistance prevents proper sugar utilization by the cells, as sugar gets stored as fat. Because I had insulin resistance—a key factor in metabolic syndrome—I needed to avoid foods that would trigger insulin production, because my body would store the energy as fat rather than burning it. I could also address insulin resistance with certain types of exercise.

Cortisol was another key hormone I had to pay attention to. Cortisol is the stress hormone that helps regulate blood pressure and the immune system during a sudden crisis. What does that have to do with diet and fitness? Cortisol is great for surviving a true crisis, but in the stress of day-to-day situations, it tells the body to eat something with a lot of calories. Cortisol is also positively influenced by diet and exercise. It was the second marker on my checklist.

Insulin and cortisol don't actually show up on blood tests. But the other numbers are clues that they're high, because they go hand in hand with the other blood markers. So if your numbers are out of range, you can count on your insulin production and cortisol levels being high.

THE MEASUREMENT BENCHMARKS—EVERY MONTH

Like a tailor, it is time to take the measuring tape and measure your waist, right around the belly button. This will tell you the adipose fat—which is the storage kind. The American Heart Association recommends that waist circumference be less than forty inches for men and thirty-five inches for women. Numbers over this value put you in a category of risk for metabolic syndrome.

MEASURE YOUR WAIST CIRCUMFERENCE

With a tape measure, start at the top of your hip bone and pull the measure around your body, level with your belly button.

A second measurement, called the waist-hip ratio, is also helpful in determining whether you're carrying weight around your waist that can be harmful to your health and keep you from being a Fat-Burning Machine. The National Institute of Diabetes and Digestive and Kidney Diseases (NIDDK) states that women with waist-hip ratios of more than 0.8, and men with more than 1.0, are at increased health risk because of their fat distribution.

MEASURE YOUR WAIST-HIP RATIO

To measure your waist-hip ratio, take a tape measure and place it around your hips at the widest point. Then place it around your waist at the narrowest point (usually above the belly button). Divide the waist circumference by the hip circumference.

WEIGHT BENCHMARKS—EVERY WEEK

If you're grimacing at the idea of regular weigh-ins and if, like me, you've experienced the tyranny of the scale, I'd like to ease your mind about it. Believe me, I used to hate the scale and I wondered why it had so much power over me. The scale doesn't have feelings. The scale is not benevolent or cruel. The scale isn't judgmental. You step on it. It gives you a number. Nothing more, nothing less. The scale is an inanimate object. And yet, the power it had over me was incredible. It could take me to the highest of highs and the lowest of lows. My relationship with this inanimate object was an emotional roller coaster of love and hate.

It seems like scales are everywhere. They are in every house I have stayed at, every hotel room, every gym, and every doctor's office. You can't really get away from them. Who could possibly use so many scales? I always thought that scales must be for other people. They weren't for people like me. How could they be? They just reminded me of things that were not going well in my life. Who would want to step on a scale?

My dysfunctional relationship with the scale started at a young age. When I was thirteen years old, I played tackle football on a traveling team. At that time, there were different positions that players were eligible to play based on their weight. Players under 135 pounds were eligible to play all positions. Players over 135 pounds could only play on the offensive or defensive line. I wanted to play cornerback. The problem was that I weighed 142 pounds.

It was such a struggle. Each week, I would have to lose about seven pounds before the game. There was no good way to lose weight as a teenager, particularly back then. My parents were clueless about how to help me, so my strategy was to basically eat normally until Friday, starve myself on Saturday and Sunday, sweat all Saturday night in heavy clothes and blankets, and then weigh in Sunday morning. I would eat candy bars to get energy before the game. As stupid as that sounds, that is what I did, and everyone thought it was pretty effective. I constantly had to weigh myself to see how tough the weight loss would be the next week. The scale was a monster, a source of dread, deciding whether I would play cornerback or not.

As I think about it, though, I didn't always have a bad relationship with my scale. I did love my scale when I was on a diet. When I was in the early success phase of a diet, I loved the scale. I weighed myself everywhere I could. At home, on the road, and even when I visited friends' houses. I remember the excitement of anticipating what *their* scales would say. It was so exhilarating. Maybe I would weigh less. When I was on a diet, my weight was dropping and I loved weighing myself every day.

Sometimes, if I was really excited about my diet and things were going well, I would even buy a new scale. As the technology changed, I bought fancy digital scales that provided all sorts of numbers—body fat percentage, BMI, etc. I didn't know how to use the scale or what the numbers really meant, but it was so much fun. I even had a weigh-in ritual. Always in the morning. Always naked. Even better if I weighed myself after exercising and before I drank a glass of water. Every little bit counts, right? My weight would be nice and low.

Those moments of happiness with my scale didn't last long. A few weeks. Maybe a month or two. Nothing longer. And then I was back to avoidance.

If I dared to weigh myself in one of the off periods, I would always weigh more than I did before my last diet. It was so frustrating, as my set point kept moving up. It never failed.

One of those fancy scales that I bought during one of my diets was a Withings Internet scale. What was so interesting about it was that it linked through Wi-Fi to my iPad. When I weighed myself, the result would instantly show up in the iPad Scale app. Now today that sounds pretty common, but five years ago, it was cutting-edge. The importance of this innovation was that I could now track my weight and the data stayed forever. It was no longer just my memory or my annual visit to the doctor's office. I could see the data, the trend lines. Every time I weighed myself, the data point showed up on the screen. It never went away. It was a mind-opening window to my life.

My Withings scale may have saved my life. I am extremely data driven, and I could now see my weight problem in a way that I could relate to. I could see my weight at a level that I didn't think was sustainable. I was on the way to 300 pounds rather than my bucket-list goal of 200 pounds. Something had to change.

The first thing to change was my relationship with my scale. I realized that my scale was a tool, just like my computer, my iPad, or my cell phone. It was time to stop projecting my emotions onto my scale. I learned to appreciate how helpful it could be to understand my weight. Looking at trend lines made a big difference. I didn't have to worry if I was up or down a couple of pounds (that could be just water weight or time of day). The point was the trend and what it meant. If I was moving up, what was I doing that I needed to stop? If I was going down, what could I learn?

> The first thing to change was my relationship with my scale. I realized that my scale was a tool, just like my computer, my iPad, or my cell phone. It was time to stop projecting my emotions onto my scale. I learned to appreciate how helpful it could be to understand my weight.

My scale was providing me reconnaissance on my body. In military reconnaissance, you watch a beachhead and nine out of ten times nothing changes. But, on that tenth time, you see movement and you have a point of reference to know what changed, how it changed, and what it means. That's what the scale was doing for me.

My scale allowed me to have a better awareness and understanding of the changes in my body. Tracking the data, I could reflect on its meaning and then make decisions going forward.

Similarly, there was no reason to obsess anymore about weighing myself constantly when things were going well. Data is data. I use it to make informed decisions. The satisfaction and fulfillment had to come from within me, not from the scale. Sometimes that fulfillment could come from clothes that fit better, a compliment from a friend, or my performance in a race.

My scale was only as powerful as I allowed it to be. For me, I just needed the facts. Nothing more. Nothing less.

Daily weigh-ins give you ongoing data, capped with a weekly "official" weigh-in. As you weigh yourself each day, think of the scale as a data-mining tool. Here's a tip: One of the hallmarks of good research is to keep as many factors as possible constant so that you can measure true change. When weighing yourself, this means keeping as many factors as possible the same—the time of day, day of the week, and clothing—so you can understand what has really changed.

> The scale doesn't have feelings. The scale is not benevolent or cruel. The scale isn't judgmental. You step on it. It gives you a number. Nothing more, nothing less.

My official weigh-in time is typically Saturday morning before breakfast. I like it because I know I will be home, I can keep it to roughly the same time, and then I can enjoy my weekend. Pick the time that works best for you.

START A FAT-BURNING JOURNAL

Becoming a Fat-Burning Machine is a conscious decision. You can't just *hope* to become one. You have to work for it. It requires you to become more familiar with your metrics and understand what drives them. What are you eating? How are you exercising? What are the weaknesses that have undermined your efforts in the past?

That's why it's important to start keeping a daily food journal of exactly what you eat—I mean everything—so that you are accountable to yourself. Once you know what you are actually eating—the food, the quantity, and the frequency—you will be able to understand the likely outcome you can expect.

I learned the importance of this journal and awareness when I started working toward becoming a Fat-Burning Machine. I know it sounds really basic, but I did not know in detail what I ate each day and I didn't keep track of my physical activity.

I could remember the big picture of my meals—oatmeal for breakfast or a steak for dinner—but I had little memory of the details. So I used the note pad function in my iPhone to start a basic journal. No big fancy chart—just writing down after each meal or at the end of the day everything that I ate and drank.

As I went through the day writing things down, I was truly shocked by what I saw. It was a reality check on how unaware I'd been. How could I possibly drink so many Diet Cokes? Did I really eat three apples at work? I was just drinking a soda or having a piece of fruit. Harmless, right? Not really. I also found that I was forgetting the food I ate that was having the biggest impact on me. The late-night snack, the handful of chips, the extra spoonfuls that weren't even conscious. Too much mindless eating.

As I looked over a week or even a specific day, I could see types of food that would turn my Fat-Burning Machine off. And one by one, I would consciously eliminate them from my diet.

I admit that at first it was really hard for me to be honest with myself. I didn't want to acknowledge some of the bad decisions I had made throughout the day. But it really helped. I could see patterns. I began to recognize situations that I would be in and it helped me anticipate my eating. Was I going to be in an airport? At a client meeting? Maybe at a hockey game? Awareness gave me a way to plan ahead.

I had to do the same thing with my fitness. I was disturbed to find that I exercised in my mind much more than I did in reality. My intentions were great, but my reality was quite sad. And when I did exercise, it didn't really help me become a Fat-Burning Machine. I equated fat burning with sweating, so I ran, which was really challenging. I often found more reasons that I couldn't run than why I could.

So in your exercise journal, record the actual exercise you did. How long did you do it? How did you feel afterward? Did you do everything that you wanted? Could you have done more? What were the limiting factors? Small notes to yourself as close to real time as possible will help you understand the outcome that you got that week.

The data in your food and exercise journal will give you all the information that you need to determine if your Fat-Burning Machine is turned on or off. The journal doesn't have to be complicated. Keep the list on your smartphone or use a blank notebook. Start with the day and just write in sequential order what you ate and any exercise or fitness activities you did that day. At the end of the day, look at what you did and reflect. Rate yourself on a one-to-five scale, with a one meaning that it was a disaster of a day and a five meaning that it was perfect.

At the end of the week, after your official weigh-in, check your daily scales to see how many days you have in the four to five range and how many days are one and two. Analyze what you ate and compare it with what you weigh. Did you get the outcome that you expected? Does your weight reflect your effort?

In their totality, these measures will keep you focused on your reality and your goal. They're the calibrations of your Fat-Burning Machine. Next, let's delve into the secrets that will make everything work.

SEVEN

AN INTRODUCTION TO THE FAT-BURNING DIET

Strategies to Sync Nutrition with Exercise

Marcela and I have been married for twenty-five years. For the first twenty years or so, before I became a Fat-Burning Machine, we did not eat the same foods. It was a constant source of frustration and angst. I liked to eat pasta, rice, pizza, steak, hot dogs, big stuffed sandwiches, and rich desserts. Marcela liked to eat salads, vegetables, fish, and chicken. She would chop up cucumbers and carrots for the kids. She made homemade soups for us in the winter and beautiful fruit salads in the summer. She never ate unhealthy, processed food. She loved almonds, Greek yogurt, and a variety of seeds.

So while our children were growing up, we had three different meals at dinner: one for me, one for Marcela, and one for the kids, which was some combination of mine and Marcela's. It was frustrating and a waste of time and money. Looking back, I can't believe it, but that was our life.

Now we all eat the same meal. The kids love Marcela's grilled shrimp on the barbecue, her delicious salads made with fresh vegetables, and her succulent grilled salmon and sliced chicken. Marcela and our daughter, Isabella, enjoy hummus with sliced vegetables as an appetizer. Our diets are mostly in sync, and they favor Marcela's natural way of eating. Long into our marriage, I've come around to what Marcela understood all along.

Being a Fat-Burning Machine has transformed my relationship with food—from mindless indulgence to making mindful choices that are not only delicious but also designed for fat burning.

A DAY IN THE LIFE OF MIKE

My breakfast routine, usually after morning exercise, doesn't deviate much from day to day. Although we'll provide a number of options in the diet, I personally prefer my go-to choice of an egg white omelet with peppers, tomato, mushrooms, and cheddar cheese. I also enjoy having a piece of whole-wheat toast. If I am particularly hungry, I will add cottage cheese. I am not a big coffee drinker. I try to drink water or iced tea with breakfast. This is the meal that gets my day started on the right track.

I take the subway to work each morning. It's a short fifteen-minute ride to my office. I work in an open space at a stand-up desk. I don't stand all day for the exercise. I stand because I find that if I sit, my muscles start to cramp up and it is actually quite uncomfortable. I also have a Bosu ball that I sometimes stand on for stabilization exercises. The Bosu ball is the perfect complement to a very long, boring conference call.

I typically have a midmorning snack at 11:00 a.m., which consists of Greek yogurt and a high-fiber snack. This keeps me going until lunch. If I am on the road, I will eat a high-fiber snack or a handful of almonds. Going into lunch hungry is always a risk for me, particularly because I often eat lunch out, with many meal choices. I usually have one of three lunch scenarios:

1. Desk lunch. My typical lunch, which is eaten at my desk, is usually a chopped salad with chicken and oil and vinegar dressing on the side.

2. Lunch out at a good-but-nothing-special restaurant. In these types of places, I am usually traveling. In this situation, I will seek out a salad of some sort or make my own. These restaurants pose the biggest risk for me because they have so many choices and, if I am hungry, I may be tempted to try something new or off-plan that could set me back for the rest of the day.

3. Lunch out at an amazing restaurant where I really want to enjoy the food. This happens once a week. I go to an incredible restaurant where the food is unique and delicious. I am more likely to take a chance and order something new and amazing. Sometimes it can be Japanese or the latest farm-to-table restaurant.

Regardless of restaurant, I have five tactics that I always use so that I can enjoy the specialty of the food, but not deviate from the plan:

1. I never go to lunch starving.

2. If I eat a salad, I will always have the dressing on the side and dip my fork before taking a bite.

3. I am not tempted by the bread, no matter how appetizing it looks. I know what bread tastes like. I don't need it.

4. I know I can't stop at one French fry, so why start?

5. I skip dessert no matter how appealing. If everyone is having something, I will ask for mixed berries to be polite.

My afternoons are usually the busiest time of the day. Lots to get done. My day can also go two ways. I can make it through the day and not even have a second to grab a snack. Or . . . I can mindlessly eat and have a couple of snacks. Neither is particularly good. Planning ahead for snacks is crucial. I am always hungry in the afternoon, particularly between 4:00 and 6:00. To avoid going to dinner hungry, I like to have a Greek yogurt and high-fiber snack before I get home.

Just because it is the last meal, it doesn't mean that dinner has to be the biggest meal of the day. It is actually when I am the most careful. Marcela and I like to cook. We have a routine—I chop and prep, she cooks, and we jointly clean the dishes.

That's my general schedule—a day in the life of Mike. But as my nine million frequent flier miles will attest, I travel a lot. I mention this to make the point that I don't really have what you could call a life routine. I spend a lot of time on the road and in hotel rooms. I eat out a lot. I have a fair amount of control over what I eat, but timing and location is quite random.

I know many people believe that having a complicated life and a busy career are the death knells of a healthy diet. Yet because there is so much uncertainty in my life routine, I have been able to use my nutrition and fitness as a way to have some continuity. No matter where I am, what time zone I am in, or what I am doing, I find ways to keep what I eat and when I work out pretty constant.

Believe it or not, following my diet on the road can actually be easier. I know that most people feel the opposite way, but without the possibility of grazing in the kitchen, I can usually stay more in control. I am not one to like going to late-night dinners or staying out all night. If I am going to functions or events, I will usually eat a premeal at my hotel. I have found that there are two global meals that anyone can make and are usually pretty healthy:

1. Egg white omelet with cheddar cheese, veggies, and ham, with wheat toast. This can be ordered just about anywhere I travel. I always specify to prepare with Pam and not oil. If I am feeling particularly hungry, I will try to get a side of cottage cheese. I try to eat a large breakfast because the rest of the day can be tricky and less predictable.

2. Mixed green salad with grilled chicken and oil and balsamic vinegar dressing on the side. You can get it anywhere and while the composition of a green salad may change, it is consistent enough. If I am particularly hungry, I will order double chicken. This is a

very good meal to order from room service, and I will usually eat it when I am going to an event that will have passed hors d'oeuvres and a set menu.

When I travel, I also bring along some emergency items like bars and a bag or two of fiber cereal. I find that they are filling and can keep me from being hungry.

Because I am so in tune with my own hunger signals and energy needs, I wanted to make sure that the Fat-Burning Machine Diet was responsive to the way people actually live and eat.

A DIET IN SYNC

At the start of my journey, I had a split personality. On one side, I was getting advice from Dr. Lefkowitz about what to eat to overcome metabolic syndrome. On the other side, I was training with Coach Mike and downing high-sugar gels, drinks, and bars that were setting me back in my weight loss efforts. When I started working with Gale, it hit me: Everything had to be in sync. Exercise alone will not turn you into a Fat-Burning Machine—you have to change your diet if you want to beat metabolic syndrome.

In fact, the more exercise I did before I changed my nutrition, the hungrier I wasn't and I was gaining weight. Eating a diet that is high in carbohydrates, even if it is only done during exercise situations, would cause my metabolic syndrome to make me a fat-storing machine, in spite of the fact that I was exercising.

This understanding was particularly meaningful because the conventional advice for sports nutrition was dead wrong. No wonder I was gaining weight while running marathons!

Syncing your nutrition to your training program will make you a Fat-Burning Machine faster. If your nutrition and training are not synced, it is like running your engine with the choke on. When they are synced, you will be a smooth-running Fat-Burning Machine.

SOME QUICK TIPS

Gale and I designed the Fat-Burning Machine diet to be full of variety and rich in the foods your body needs. Your body needs carbohydrates, fat, and protein in order to survive. But not all carbohydrates, fats, and proteins are created equally. The carbohydrates contained in vegetables are different from those contained in a muffin or orange juice. Your orange juice may be far from healthy. As a quick guide, choose from the list of fat-burning foods and avoid the fat-storing foods in the chart below. That doesn't mean you can never have the foods in the fat-storing column. They're just not your best choices. On page 79 you'll find a full list of fat-burning foods to incorporate into your diet and lots of suggestions for making delicious meals.

Top Fat-STORING Foods

Breaded or fried meats

Chicken nuggets, chicken-fried steak

Breaded or fried fish or seafood

Fish and chips

Processed foods, like frozen meals

Sweet-and-sour meat, seafood, vegetables

Pasta or pizza

Spaghetti and marinara or Alfredo sauce

Calzone, stromboli

Potpies (turkey, chicken, beef, salmon)

Sweet and spicy wings

Baked beans with honey or brown sugar

Pastries and baked goods made with refined flour and sugar—cakes, pies, cookies, brownies

Muffins, scones

Bread and crackers made with refined flour

Bagels, croissants

Pancakes, waffles, French toast

Sweetened granola, granola bars

Boxed cereal

Canned soups or vegetables with added sugar

Refried beans with added fat

Biscuits and gravy, stuffing

Prepared sauces containing sugar

Any foods or oils containing the words "hydrogenated" or "partially hydrogenated"

Margarine

Artificial cheese

Potatoes, French fries, tater tots

Onion rings

Top Fat-STORING Foods (continued)

Corn

Chowders—corn, clam, crab

Popcorn, corn, potato, and "snack" chips

Trail mix (sweetened or with fruit)

Fruit juice—especially orange, grapefruit, cherry, cranberry, mango, blended fruit

Fruit rolls, dried fruit

Fruit-sweetened or fruit-at-the-bottom yogurt

Sugar

*Artificial sweeteners

Honey, maple syrup, agave

All foods containing the words "sucrose," "dextrose," "glucose," "galactose," "maltose," or any word ending in "ose"

Any food containing high-fructose corn syrup or corn syrup solids

Foods containing any type of added sugar, syrup, molasses, caramel, malt, and maltodextrin

Foods containing names like muscovado, diatase, treacle, evaporated cane juice, and fruit juice concentrate

Soda (sugared and diet)

High-sugar condiments—ketchup, barbecue sauce, steak sauce

Pickle relish

Hollandaise sauce

Jams and jellies

Bottled salad dressings with sugar

Candy

Ice cream, frozen yogurt, sherbet

Popsicles (sugared)

Whipped cream

Chocolate sauce

Sugared coffee drinks, sweet tea, cocoa

Energy drinks

Milk shakes, malts

Beer, wine, and alcohol

* occasional use only—one to two servings per week

Top Fat-BURNING Foods

Fresh vegetables, especially dark leafy greens (spinach, kale, collard greens), asparagus, Brussels sprouts, broccoli, cauliflower, peppers, squash [see page 93]

Fresh meat—beef, chicken, lamb, pork, venison, buffalo

Beef or turkey jerky

Cured and deli meat—ham, sausage, bacon, smoked turkey

Chicken and poultry—chicken, duck, goose, quail, turkey

Seafood and fish (all)— [see page 92]

Smoked fish

Canned tuna, anchovies, sardines

Tofu

Plain Greek yogurt and other plain yogurt

Cheese (all)—cow, goat, hard, soft

Cottage cheese

Cream cheese

Ricotta cheese

Eggs

Egg whites (carton)

* Fruit—low-to-moderate-sugar varieties, such as apple, avocado, blackberry, blueberry, cantaloupe, coconut, cranberry, lemon, lime, peach, raspberry, strawberry, rhubarb, watermelon

Vegetable oils—olive, canola, coconut, sesame, sunflower, walnut

Butter

Nut butters (unsugared)—peanut, almond, cashew, sesame, sunflower

Mayonnaise

Milk—cow, almond, soy, coconut, rice

Nuts and seeds, such as almonds, walnuts, cashews, macadamias, pecans, chickpeas, pumpkin seeds, sesame seeds, sunflower seeds

Vinegar

Mustard

Hummus

Salsa

Tahini

Sriracha

Soy sauce, tamari

Pesto

** High-fiber whole grains, such as oatmeal, rice, rice cakes, whole-grain bread, rye crisp, flaxseed bread and crackers, and quinoa

** Fresh beans and peas

** Canned, unsweetened beans

Sugar-free coffee and tea

Herbs

All spices and (unsugared) dry seasonings

* in moderation—one serving per day or less
** in moderation—choice of one to two servings per day of beans, peas, or grains as shown on menus in Chapter Eight.

You've been misled that fat is bad. It is not. Fat can provide energy and improve health markers. However, fat in combination with highly refined carbohydrates or plain sugar turns off fat burning and destroys your health markers. Be knowledgeable about the *types* of fat in your diet. Avoid foods with trans fats or partially hydrogenated fats—in other words, most processed foods. Saturated fats in meat and poultry can be eaten in moderation, but choose the leaner cuts of meat. White meat chicken and turkey are less fatty than beef and venison, especially the breast meat. Healthy omega-3 fatty acids in fish (especially salmon, trout, catfish, and mackerel) make them excellent fat-burners. Olive oil and avocados both contain monounsaturated fat, which is considered heart healthy. Nuts and seeds, especially walnuts, almonds, and sesame, pumpkin, and sunflower seeds, are excellent sources of protein, but should be eaten in moderation because of their high calorie count. This diet is somewhat higher in fat than many, but it favors the "good" fats that promote fat burning. But be aware of this: High-fat breaded and fried foods are not what we mean by good fat. Pan-fry and sauté using healthy oil like olive, coconut, or canola oil. On this plan, butter is also OK. When you cook with regular butter, you'll get more flavor, but it will burn at a lower temperature and more quickly than other fats due to the presence of milk solids, so clarified butter is more fit for this use.

Too much fruit encourages fat storage. Fruit should be a treat and not a staple. Choose fruits from the low-sugar varieties.

HIGH- AND LOW-SUGAR FRUITS		
HIGH-Sugar Fruits (Avoid)	MEDIUM-Sugar Fruits (Eat very occasionally)	LOW-Sugar Fruits (Enjoy, but don't overdo)
Banana	Apple	Avocado
Cherries	Blueberries	Blackberries
Grapes	Cantaloupe	Cranberries
Kiwi	Peach	Raspberries
Mango	Strawberries	Lemon
Orange	Watermelon	Lime
Pear		Rhubarb
Pineapple		
Plum		
Tangerine		

Finally, a word about fiber. The vegetables in the diet are high in fiber, but if you're in situations where they're not easy to come by, you might need to have limited amounts of high-fiber grains, such as brown rice, oatmeal, and quinoa, along with beans and peas. Fiber is known to be a significant factor in reversing metabolic syndrome and fighting obesity. Just watch the amounts.

A GLASS OF WINE WITH DINNER?

One of the most common questions our fat-burners ask is whether or not they can have a glass of wine with dinner or a drink after work. Our answer: Do what you like, but know the facts. The current research is that moderate alcohol consumption actually improves cardiovascular health—moderate being defined as one drink a day for women and two drinks for men. But even if that's the case, it's not the whole story. Drinking can also stall weight loss. Studies show that fat burning and metabolism are affected for twenty-five to forty-eight hours after alcohol consumption. There is also an increased risk of problems when combining exercise and alcohol. If you like to go out for a drink after playing sports, it could have an extra negative effect, since your blood sugar naturally drops during exercise and your body is working on replacing your glycogen stores once you are finished. Consuming alcohol during this time will halt this process and can cause blood sugar levels to stay at an unhealthy level.

If you do drink, be careful; that's when bad decision-making can happen. Don't sabotage the good work you're doing. Stick with a glass of dry red or white wine (5 ounces) or a spirit (1.5 ounces, without caloric mixers), and watch the portions. It's easy to over-pour! Whether you drink or not, keep your goal of being a Fat-Burning Machine at the top of your priority list and ask yourself whether that drink is furthering your goal or impeding it. Take a week or two off from alcohol at the beginning of the diet and check out how you feel. Or if you usually have a drink every day and don't want to give it up altogether, try reducing your intake to one to three times a week. Nurse a drink throughout the evening with a side of water. And when you do drink, enjoy it. Don't waste the calories on the cheap stuff. Embrace and own your choices.

IN YOUR PANTRY

Stock the following essentials for fat-burners in your fridge and pantry at all times. You can always whip up something with these basics.

Staples: Olive oil, canola oil, coconut oil, sea salt, pepper, white vinegar, balsamic vinegar, mustard, fresh herbs, and spices to taste.

Basic Vegetables: Red and white onions; garlic; spinach; kale; carrots; celery; red, green, and yellow bell peppers; leeks; zucchini; lettuce; tomatoes; carrots.

Protein: Eggs, chicken, meat (beef, ham, lamb, pork, venison, poultry), smoked salmon, fish, tofu, canned tuna, sliced deli meats.

Dairy: Yogurt (preferably Greek), cheese, cottage cheese.

Grains: High-fiber cereal, oatmeal, low-carb crackers, quinoa.

Fruit: Lemons, limes (and their juices), variety of low-sugar fruits of personal choice.

Nuts and seeds: Almonds, walnuts, cashews, macadamias, pecans, pumpkin seeds, sesame seeds, sunflower seeds.

Why Greek Yogurt Is Better

You've noticed that I always specify Greek yogurt. It's preferable for fat burning because it's made using a different process from other yogurts. As a result, it has twice the protein and half the carbs of regular yogurt. It also tastes great.

Gale, who spends her life training athletes, pointed out to me that training isn't just about exercise. It's also about nutrition. That's exactly what we're doing with the Fat-Burning Machine Diet. We're helping you with a nutrition training plan that you can enjoy for the rest of your life.

GALE TALKS ABOUT HUNGER

Everyone embarking on a new diet plan has one big fear: hunger. Pause for a moment and think about what it feels like to be hungry. Can you describe it? How do you feel when you're hungry? Notice this feeling is different than when you feel other emotions.

With our approach of eating three meals and two or three snacks per day, we keep you from getting really hungry. The point of this program is not to see how much willpower you do or don't have. We want to prevent trouble before it is an issue. Why? Because hungry people do stupid and emotional things that sabotage success. In desperation to feel better, they eat unhealthy foods and purchase unhealthy items at the grocery store. We don't want you to feel starving, ravenous, and desperate. We want you to be satisfied with good, nutritious foods.

That process starts with identifying *why* you are eating before you eat.

Feeling hungry and eating because you're hungry is different from eating because you are tired, stressed, bored, thirsty, anxious, or you eat simply out of habit at a particular time of the day.

Some of us eat when we feel stress. We want something, anything, to make the stress go away. Eating a pint of ice cream doesn't make the stress go away, but it sure feels good to the mouth and senses for a small amount of time. Instant pleasure, ahhhh . . .

That instant gratification isn't long lasting. For most people, there is a feeling of regret and sadness, especially after consuming too much of a sugary food. Many people feel an instant high shortly after consuming the food, and within a short amount of time there is a low, tired feeling. This crashing feeling is the blood sugar high, then the insulin spike, shortly followed by a blood sugar low. Then you eat something sweet again to feel good again. This is a chemical chain reaction in your body with disastrous effects.

Sounds like drug addition, doesn't it? Studies have shown that people can and do exhibit addictive behaviors with sugar. One study found that sugar can even be more rewarding than addictive drugs. What? Sugar is more addictive than cocaine? Yes.

Removing as much sugar from your diet as possible will help you succeed. Not only will you feel better, you will feel more in control of your eating and your emotions. Furthermore, getting sugar out of your diet will help your blood markers improve. And the best reason for removing sugar from your diet? It forces your body to access fat for fuel.

Recognize that training your mind to be aware of emotional eating takes time. You will have failures from time to time. All of that is part of the process. As long as you are generally—80 percent of the time—heading in the right direction, feel good about yourself. Aiming for 100 percent perfection is a recipe for heartbreak and failure. Allow for self-correction and "getting back on your game" after an occasional misstep.

SET YOURSELF UP FOR SUCCESS

Before making changes to your diet, set yourself up for success. Get rid of all the sweet, sugary snacks in your house and in your office drawers. Take the cookies to work and share them with people that are not interested in becoming a Fat-Burning Machine. They are happy and you don't have to waste food.

Have foods prepared and readily available that you can easily access when you're hungry and need a snack. For example, take one night of the week to clean and cut vegetables. Measure out quarter- or half-cup servings of nuts and put the portions in snack bags. Carry the

RETRAINING YOUR BRAIN TO LOVE HEALTHY FOOD

By Dr. Laura Lefkowitz

Many people tell me they just can't change their diets because they lack the willpower. When I delve deeper, they are really saying that healthy foods don't taste good to them, while their favorite rich, creamy, fatty foods do. Faced with the choice between a plate of fresh zucchini and a plate of French fries, only the French fries get them salivating. This response is absolutely normal when you've been conditioned by a lifetime of responding to certain food cues. For example, when I see the colors orange and pink together, I have a physical craving for doughnuts and coffee. Those colors together trigger my brain to think about Dunkin Donuts, a place I frequented my entire childhood. That is how strong the neural response of conditioning can be. You don't even have to see a doughnut to crave it—just images that hint at a doughnut can cause a craving/salivating response.

snack bags in your purse or car console, or store them in a small cooler in your car or office. (There is a large selection of snack suggestions in Chapter Eight.)

Plan ahead for social events. There will be times when you are invited to a social gathering that you know will be a fat-storing event. Eat a small salad or some vegetables before the event, if possible, so you can keep portion sizes small. Enjoy the food, enjoy the people at the event, and get back to your new routine tomorrow. Again, as long as you're following the guidelines most of the time, you will have success.

Every child is born with a blank slate of emotions and responses toward food, but the conditioning process starts from their first taste of breast milk or formula. Humans evolved with primitive responses that favor sweet and fatty foods for survival, because these foods indicated caloric content and therefore ensured survival in the harsh elements. But in modern times of shelter, heat, air conditioning, cars, and supermarkets packed with an abundance of food, these primitive proclivities are causing an obesity epidemic.

If you're a hungry child and your parents respond with doughnuts, hot dogs, and rich pasta dishes, you will eventually salivate when you see those foods. When you see foods like lettuce and kale, you'll have a negative response because your brain is so attuned to the *taste and texture* of sweet, fatty, oily, creamy types of food that you've been conditioned to love. Eventually, that conditioning is set, which is why so many people find healthy foods unappealing.

Now you're in a situation where eating all the food that you love has made you overweight and unhealthy. It's not about going on and off diets; it's about changing the way your brain responds to food. You have to decondition yourself. The good news is that your brain is flexible like plastic—it can change. This is referred to as neuroplasticity. If you remove unhealthy stimuli from your environment (doughnuts, pizza, Alfredo sauce, etc.) and bombard it with a new environment of healthy stimuli, the brain will adapt to this new environment. I developed this concept, which I call "Palate Training"—although the actual training takes place in your brain. Your brain will actually start to register vegetables and lean protein as palatable, enjoyable foods.

When you first decide to change your diet, you might eat a kale salad and complain, "It's like eating grass." But through repeated exposure, you will start to retrain your palate. In time your brain will get the message that healthy foods offer a reward—weight loss, more energy, and/or a better self-image. Your palate will begin to respond positively to the taste of kale salad.

This process does not happen instantly, but every time you make a behavior change, your neurons are recording the new conditioning and establishing new pathways. Your brain changes a little bit with each action. The more often you repeat the action, the more quickly your conditioning will change. A new, healthy type of memory is formed in the brain's hippocampus. Over time you can literally retrain your brain to find pleasure in a food you once would have considered tasteless or unappealing.

In my experience there are levels of change. There is a pre-contemplation phase where you are not consciously aware that you want to change, but subconsciously there is a desire for change. Then there is the contemplation phase, when you are thinking about changing, but you are not ready to commit. And then there are the action phases, where true change occurs. Unfortunately, when it comes to weight loss, doing a little bit is not that effective. Reconditioning will only happen if you do it repeatedly over time. People fail when they do a little here and there and are inconsistent. They also fail when they try to trick the brain. Diet plans based on so-called healthier versions of junk food—for example, diet brownies—don't work because the brain is still responding to brownies. It doesn't record the difference that, "These brownies are made with honey and whole-wheat flour." All the brain sees is a sweet, gooey brownie.

How do you know that your Palate Training is working? I look for these three signs.

1. You stop feeling regret over what you are not eating. You lose the "woe is me" attitude. Instead of moaning, "Everyone was eating cake and I couldn't have it," you say "I'm so proud of myself. Everyone was eating cake and I didn't have any."

2. You have a boost in confidence. When you begin looking and feeling good, you realize that all of your efforts have been worthwhile. Maybe you're fitting into a smaller clothing size. Maybe people are complimenting you. These are real, measurable rewards that get processed in the brain and reinforce your Palate Training for healthier foods.

3. You feel that you are in control of your actions. You are no longer afraid of that nefarious enemy "willpower." If you're going on a trip or out to a nice restaurant, you no longer fear that you'll lose control. You are able to plan in advance for success.

Eating well is an ideal that is grounded for life. If you view it as a loss, as a thing of regret, you cannot be successful. If you are always looking ahead to the moment when you can return to your old conditioning, you will never be successful. Success comes from experiencing genuine pleasure in eating the foods that will make you healthy and fit. There is no need to worry about willpower when you have *brain*power.

THE THREE MOST IMPORTANT THINGS TO DO

One of our beginner fat-burners asked, "Can you tell me the most important things I need to know to succeed?" Here is our list.

Adhere to the morning meal guidelines. Eating a breakfast that is high in protein and fat with moderate to low carbohydrates forces your body to use fat for fuel. Keeping insulin levels in check helps control appetite as well. If you're used to skipping breakfast and then being ravenous midmorning, this isn't helping you. We want to keep your blood sugars and appetite under control.

Snack. Too often, people don't plan to snack or they don't have a snack handy. A low-sugar snack can help prevent you from being as hungry as a lion come dinnertime. Eating snacks with the appropriate macronutrient (carbohydrate, fat, and protein) balance will keep insulin levels in check and prevent low blood sugar. When blood sugar is stabilized, the body releases insulin to utilize food as fuel, rather than to store it as fat. Exercise combined with the wrong food choices causes hunger, stunts insulin release, and encourages fat storage.

Adhere to the evening meal guidelines. We are training your body to use fat for fuel, rather than preferentially using readily available sugar. While you're busy sleeping, it's a good time to build fat for fuel. Avoid sugary after-dinner treats. A great tip from one of our fat-burners is to finish dinner, floss your teeth, and brush them. This mouth cleaning helps prevent him from having a desire to eat more food late at night. See if his tip helps you.

EIGHT

THE FAT-BURNING MACHINE DIET

The High-octane Food Plan

In the Fat-Burning Machine Diet, we blend foods that go together to burn fat rather than store it. When you first look at this plan, it will look like a diet. Maybe some of the choices feel strange. Different from what you eat now, requiring a change in your habits. That's OK. If you didn't need to change, you wouldn't be here.

But what you need to know is that these are not "diet" foods. They are just different from what you probably eat now. And as your body and brain adjust, you will get the same pleasure and sensations from these meals that you get from the meals that you currently eat.

So have a little faith. Stick with them for a little while before you judge and you will see that the tastes, sensations, and feelings that you get from these meals will be the same or even better than what you are eating now. Anecdotally, I will tell you that we hear that our high-octane foods burn so smoothly that people report more energy and feeling lighter on their feet.

THE FAT-BURNING MACHINE DIET FORMULA

Let's start with the basics. A simple Fat-Burning Machine Diet formula will help you make the right choices. Whether you're designing your own meals, using one of our menu plans, or dining out, this formula should serve as your guide:

1. Select a protein option—meat, poultry, fish and seafood, eggs, dairy, or tofu. As a general rule, eat portion sizes of four to six ounces at breakfast and lunch, and six to eight ounces at dinner. Grill, roast, steam, or sauté. In this category, choose:

FISH	SHELLFISH	POULTRY	MEAT
Catfish	Clams	Chicken	Beef
Cod	Crab	Chicken eggs	Ham
Flounder	Crayfish	Duck	Lamb
Halibut	Lobster	Duck eggs	Pork
Haddock	Mussels	Goose	Venison
Herring	Oysters	Goose eggs	
Mackerel	Squid	Quail	
Salmon	Scallops	Quail eggs	**DAIRY**
Snapper	Shrimp	Squab	Greek yogurt
Sole		Turkey	Cheese
Striped bass			Cottage cheese
Swordfish	**CANNED FISH**		
Tilapia	Anchovies		
Tuna	Sardines		
Trout	Tuna		**TOFU**

2. Select a low-carbohydrate vegetable option. Eat an unlimited amount of green leafy and other green vegetables, and approximately one cup of red and orange vegetables. Steam, roast, or grill vegetables, or lightly sauté them in one tablespoon of olive, coconut, or canola oil, or butter. Use vegetable oil spray, if you prefer.

GREEN LEAFY VEGETABLES	GENERAL VEGETABLES	RED AND ORANGE VEGETABLES
Bok choy	Artichokes	Beets
Broccoli	Asparagus	Carrots
Collard greens	Brussels sprouts	Pumpkin
Kale	Cabbage	Squash
Lettuce (any type)	Cauliflower	Bell peppers
Mustard greens	Celery	Sweet potatoes
Spinach	Cucumbers	Tomatoes
Turnip greens	Eggplant	
	Green beans	
	Mushrooms	
	Okra	
	Zucchini	

3. Add a fat option. Your diet should contain 40 to 55 percent fat. Most of that will come from your protein option. You also have the choice of adding nuts and oils to cook or for dressings.

OILS	BUTTER	NUTS
Canola		Almonds
Coconut	MAYONNAISE	Almond milk
Olive		Cashews
Soybean		Macadamias
Sesame		Pecans
Tahini		Walnuts

4. Add a *very limited* serving size of a carbohydrate that is mostly complex with very little to zero added sugar. This category includes high-fiber snacks, low-fat granolas, and low-carb cereals, crackers, and breads. This category also includes a very limited serving size of things like rice, beans, and quinoa. The fruit choices are limited to lower-sugar options.

RICE AND GRAINS	BEANS AND PEAS	FRUIT
Amaranth	Black beans	Apple
Barley	Chickpeas	Avocado
Flax	Kidney beans	Blackberries
Oats	Lentils	Blueberries
Quinoa	Navy beans	Cantaloupe
Pumpkin seeds	Soybeans	Cranberries
Rice	Soy milk	Lemon
Sesame seeds	Split peas	Lime
Wild rice		Peaches
		Raspberries
		Rhubarb
		Strawberries
		Watermelon

A word about dressings and condiments

- Oil, vinegar, and lemon juice are always acceptable.

- The dressings in Chapter Nine have been designed for fat burning, so mix up a batch and use them.

- Good fat-burning choices are mustard, pesto, soy sauce, tahini, and hot sauce.

- Small amounts of mayonnaise or other low-sugar creamy dressings are acceptable.

- Check all bottled dressings and condiments for sugar-free variet-ies. There is even low-sugar ketchup.

- Flavor dishes with fresh herbs and spices when possible.

The following selection of sample menus will give you many new ideas of how to prepare foods in a satisfying and delicious way. Menu selections with an asterisk (*) indicate a recipe in Chapter Nine. There are also menu options for dining out at your favorite restaurants. If you prefer, you can select your own options from the lists above, using the basic meal formula. The bottom line: We want you to feel a sense of abundance with this diet, and know that you have a wide variety of choices.

NOTE: We don't count calories on this diet. The quantities given are general guidelines. We realize that people come in all sizes and you may need to increase the amounts listed or add an extra vegetable or protein. Don't overdo it, but don't leave the table hungry.

FAT-BURNING BREAKFAST MENUS

Fat-Burning Breakfast 1

HEARTY OMELET

2 whole eggs, or 1 egg with 2 egg whites

1 ounce shredded cheese

¼ cup chopped tomatoes and onions

Cook in 1 tablespoon olive oil

Carb options: 1 slice whole-wheat toast or English muffin

General options: Replace chopped tomatoes and onions with 1 grilled tomato

Replace chopped tomatoes and onions with ½ avocado

Replace cheese with 1 slice ham or 1 sausage

Replace cheese with 1 tablespoon butter for toast or English muffin

Fat-Burning Breakfast 2

*SALMON BREAKFAST SOUFFLÉ

Carb options: ½ cup berries or apple slices, or ½ cup oatmeal, or ½ cup high-fiber cereal

Fat-Burning Breakfast 3

OMEGA-3 FISH BREAKFAST

4–6 ounces fish (cod, salmon, tuna, trout, or tilapia), grilled, baked, or sautéed

1 tablespoon olive oil

1 cup fresh vegetables (such as mushrooms, broccoli, bell peppers, or onions)

1 cup whole-fat or 2% cottage cheese

Carb options: 1 apple or 1 cup cantaloupe slices, or ½ cup rice

Fat-Burning Breakfast 4

GREEK YOGURT DELIGHT

1 cup whole-fat or 2% Greek yogurt, topped with cinnamon and ¼ cup raw, unsalted nuts (almonds, walnuts, cashews, macadamias, or pecans)

Carb options: ½ cup fresh berries (blueberries, raspberries, blackberries, strawberries) or ½ cup cooked steel-cut or 5-minute oatmeal

Fat-Burning Breakfast 5

VEGGIE-EGG SCRAMBLE

2 eggs with 1 tablespoon butter or olive oil, scrambled with tomato, zucchini, onion, and green pepper

Carb options: 1 slice whole-wheat toast or ½ cup fresh berries (blueberries, raspberries, blackberries, strawberries)

General options: Choose other vegetables, such as mushrooms, spinach, or kale

Add 1 tablespoon butter for toast

Fat-Burning Breakfast 6

TRADITIONAL EGGS

2 eggs scrambled or pan-fried in 1 tablespoon olive oil

1 slice lean deli ham or Canadian bacon

½ sliced avocado

Carb options: 1 slice whole-wheat toast, ½ English muffin, ½ cup cooked quinoa, or ½ cup long-grain brown rice

General options: Replace avocado with sliced tomatoes

Replace avocado with roasted sweet potato

Add 1 tablespoon butter for toast or English muffin

Fat-Burning Breakfast 7

*STEVE'S EASY EGG WHITE SOUFFLÉ

5 roasted asparagus spears

½ sliced tomato

Carb options: 1 slice toast or ½ English muffin

General option: Add 1 tablespoon butter for toast or English muffin

Fat-Burning Breakfast 8

SAUSAGE AND KALE FRY-UP

1 egg, scrambled, with:

1 cup chopped kale

2 breakfast sausages

1 tablespoon olive or canola oil

Carb option: 1 slice whole-wheat toast

General options: Replace sausages with 2 slices thin deli ham

Replace sausages with an extra egg and egg white

Add 1 tablespoon butter for toast

Fat-Burning Breakfast 9

COTTAGE CHEESE SWIRL

1 cup whole-fat or 2% cottage cheese sprinkled with cinnamon, nutmeg, or other spices

½ to 1 cup fresh berries, diced

Carb options: 1 cup cooked steel-cut oatmeal or 1 cup high-fiber cereal

General option: Replace cottage cheese with Greek yogurt

Fat-Burning Breakfast 10

ATHLETE'S BREAKFAST

*Athlete's Omelet

Carb options: 1 slice whole-wheat toast or ½ English muffin

General options: Add ½ avocado

Add 1 tablespoon butter for toast or English muffin

Fat-Burning Breakfast 11

SMOKED SALMON PLATTER

4 ounces thinly sliced smoked salmon

2 tablespoons cream cheese

Sliced tomato

Sliced cucumber

Sliced onion

Romaine leaves

Carb option: ½ bagel

General options: Replace smoked salmon with herring

Replace cream cheese with ½ cup Greek yogurt

Fat-Burning Breakfast 12

HIGH-FIBER GUT CHECK

1 cup high-fiber cereal

1 cup Greek yogurt

Carb option: ½ cup berries

General options: Add 6 ounces vegetable juice

Replace Greek yogurt with 6 ounces soy milk

Fat-Burning Breakfast 13

TOMATO TOPPER

Grilled tomato with poached egg on top

1 slice thin deli ham

½ baked sweet potato

Carb options: ½ cup cantaloupe slices or 1 slice whole-wheat toast

General options: Replace ham with slice of deli turkey or sausage

Add 1 tablespoon butter for toast

Fat-Burning Breakfast 14

ON-THE-GO SMOOTHIE

Mix in a blender: 1 cup spinach, 1 cup kale, ½ medium bunch parsley,
the juice of one lemon, 1 scoop protein powder (optional),
ice cubes, and 4 ounces water

Carb option: Add ½ cup mixed fruit for a veggie-fruit fusion

General option: Choose your own veggies from the list provided on page 93

Fat-Burning Breakfast 15

HEALTHY BURRITO BREAKFAST

*Omelet Burrito

Carb option: ½ cup black beans

Fat-Burning Breakfast 16

LUNCH BAG BREAKFAST

*Take-and-Go Egg Cups

Carb options: ½ cup melon slices or 1 apple

Fat-Burning Breakfast 17

FILLING FRITTATA

*Asparagus and Goat Cheese Frittata

Carb options: 1 slice whole-wheat toast or ½ cup berries

General option: Add 1 tablespoon butter for toast

Tips for Breakfast Success

Breakfast is very important. You want to start your day off right as a Fat-Burning Machine. Do not skip breakfast.

- Sautéing instructions: Some people prefer to use a non-stick cooking spray and others prefer butter or olive oil. More than likely, using a nonstick spray will contribute fewer calories, but the fat in acceptable oils is good.

- Pay attention to which combinations of foods work best for you. Which combinations do you enjoy? Which foods do you not like at all? Find a routine that includes foods that taste good to you, fill you up, and give you energy. Not all of them will. Everyone is different. Also, be careful with quantities on the carb options. Stick with the guidelines.

- Give yourself at least a week to adapt to the changes in your diet. If you are not feeling better or your clothes aren't starting to fit better, make small changes. If you are having trouble losing weight, decrease the carbohydrate options for one or two weeks, as you may be more insulin resistant than others.

- Check your portion sizes. Don't under-eat. Too much calorie restriction slows metabolism. And, finally, are you skipping meals or snacks? Too many overweight people think that losing weight means skipping meals. We want you to eat five times a day to keep your hormones at a steady level.

- For an early morning workout that begins within an hour or so of getting out of bed, consume only water, tea, or coffee before the workout. No milk, sugar, or any other added sweeteners—including artificial sweeteners. Drink only water during the workout if it is less than ninety minutes long.

- If you do a morning workout, aim to eat a normal breakfast very soon after. Don't let hours go by before you eat. Your body needs the recovery fuel.

Red Flags

- Fructose, the sugar in fruit, can be a fat-storing food, especially if you are insulin resistant. For the first two weeks, avoiding fruit is a good idea, and then bring it back in.

FAT-BURNING LUNCH MENUS

Fat-Burning Lunch 1

*TURKEY BLUEBERRY SALAD

Fresh vegetable garnishes—lettuce, tomatoes, cucumbers on the side

*Vegetable Stock

Carb options: 1 small pita pocket or 1 slice whole-wheat bread

General option: Replace Vegetable Stock with another soup in Chapter Nine

Fat-Burning Lunch 2

SPINACH SALAD

Large salad with spinach, 1 sliced hard-boiled egg,
1 ounce crumbled goat cheese, cucumbers, tomatoes.
Add a choice of 4–6 ounces grilled chicken, fish, or beef to the salad.

Carb options: ½ cup fresh berries or a handful of croutons

General option: Add a handful of raw mixed nuts

Fat-Burning Lunch 3

SOUP AND SALAD

*Cauliflower Soup

Green salad or raw vegetables. Good choices include sliced bell peppers, sweet
pea pods, carrots, celery, cucumber, and broccoli.

Carb options: 1 cup watermelon pieces

*Replace salad with 1 slice deli turkey or ham on 1 slice whole-wheat bread with
mustard, lettuce, and tomato*

General option: Choose a different soup or chili from Chapter Nine menus

Fat-Burning Lunch 4

*DANIELLE'S SUPER SANDWICH

A special treat every week or two, with turkey, avocado, and tomato

General option: Add 6 ounces soy milk

Fat-Burning Lunch 5

*GRILLED SPICY SHRIMP SALAD

Carb options: 1 cup cooked long-grain brown rice or quinoa

Fat-Burning Lunch 6

ROMAINE WRAPS

Roll lean turkey, chicken, and sliced cheese of your choice in romaine leaves.

*Asian Slaw

Carb options: 1 cup barley soup

*General option: Add 1 tablespoon *Low-Sugar BBQ Sauce*

Fat-Burning Lunch 7

*SMOKED SALMON SALAD OR WRAP

Choose either the salad or the wrap.

Carb options: Add ¼ cup pumpkin or sesame seeds

General option: Add 1 cup sliced beets

Fat-Burning Lunch 8

VEGETARIAN CORNUCOPIA

*Roasted Eggplant with Raw Vegan Pesto

*Gale's Health Salad

General option: Add 6 ounces almond milk

Fat-Burning Lunch 9

SALAD NICOISE

Tuna, green beans, hard-boiled egg, tomato, bell pepper, olives, sprig of parsley

Dressing: 1 tablespoon olive oil, 2 tablespoons vinegar, 1 teaspoon dried mustard

*General option: Add 1 cup *Asparagus Soup Puree*

Fat-Burning Lunch 10

SATISFYING STEW

*Seafood Stew

Carb options: 2 rye crisps or rice cakes

Fat-Burning Lunch 11

BURGER MELT

Hamburger patty, 4–6 ounces, with melted cheese (optional)

Lettuce, tomato, onion, pickle, mustard

Carb options: ½ spelt bun

*General options: 2 tablespoons *Guacamole or ½ avocado*

Fat-Burning Lunch 12

BACON BLUE CHEESE SALAD

Bacon, lettuce, tomato, and avocado, with 2 tablespoons blue cheese dressing

*Carb options: 1 slice whole-wheat bread or spelt roll, 1 apple,
or replace with *BLT Wrap*

Fat-Burning Lunch 13

WHOLESOME MIDDAY BREAK

*Zucchini Pasta with Roasted Tomatoes & Chimichurri

*Poblano Pepper and Vegetable Chicken Soup

General option: ½ cup sugar-free Jell-O

Fat-Burning Lunch 14

CHILI BOWL

*Slow Cooker Texican Chili

Mixed green salad with vinaigrette or *Creamy Dressing

Carb options: Add ½ cup cooked kidney beans to chili

*General option: Replace chili with *Poblano White Chili or *Slow Cooker Beef and Vegetable Chili*

Fat-Burning Lunch 15

MIDDAY FAVORITE

*Ratatouille

Carb options: ½ cup rice or quinoa

General option: Top vegetables with cooked sausage

Serve with crumbled goat cheese

Fat-Burning Lunch 16

MEXICAN-STYLE FAT-BURNER

*Omelet Burrito

*Guacamole

Carb options: Add a handful of low-carb tortilla chips

Fat-Burning Lunch 17

ENERGY BOOSTER

*Poblano Pepper and Vegetable Chicken Soup

*Salmon Cilantro Salad

Carb options: 1 slice whole-wheat bread or 2 rye crisps

Tips for Lunch Success

- When setting yourself up for success as a Fat-Burning Machine, completely eliminate items with added sugar, such as ketchup, tartar sauce, etc. Just so you know, ketchup is high in sugar. One tablespoon has four grams of carbohydrates—all of which are sugar. Read the labels before consuming condiments, or use your smartphone to look up the ingredients before putting potential junk into your body.

- Be certain you are not overeating—especially cheese. Measure portions and keep a mental image of size. For example, is six ounces of meat the same size as the palm of your hand? If not, how does a six-ounce portion compare to the palm of your hand? Can you hold a quarter cup in your hand? Or is a quarter cup more or less than the cupped portion of your hand?

- Be self-aware in social lunch situations. Eat to please yourself and no one else. You control your own success. Never go to lunch hungry. Skip the bread. No bites, licks, or tastes.

- Place salad dressing on the side. Dip your fork in the dressing and take a bite of salad.

- You can use any spice you please in unlimited quantities.

Red Flags

- Don't skip your morning snack. You'll be too hungry at lunch and risk overeating.

- As much as possible, plan lunch in advance. Grabbing food on the go can be trouble.

FAT-BURNING DINNER MENUS

REMINDER: In general, avoid carb options at dinner during the 12-week plan. If you're still hungry, add a larger portion of salad and/or vegetables.

Fat-Burning Dinner 1

*CHICKEN ESQUITES

*Asian Soup with Baked Tofu

Fat-Burning Dinner 2

VEGETARIAN FAVORITE

*Asparagus Soup Puree

*Zucchini Pasta with Roasted Tomatoes & Chimichurri

Avocado and tomato slices

Fat-Burning Dinner 3

FISH OR CHICKEN GRILL

6–8 ounces grilled fish or chicken

*Spicy Fish Marinade

*Roasted Rapini or *Sautéed Greens

Green salad

Fat-Burning Dinner 4

FAVORITE CHICKEN DINNER

*Chicken Pesto Chimichurri Over Sautéed Spinach

*Roasted Brussels sprouts

Green salad

Fat-Burning Dinner 5

ASIAN STIR-FRY

Mix together 6–8 ounces of your favorite lean meat, fish, or tofu with abundant vegetables—broccoli, bell peppers, onion, snow peas, zucchini. For a heartier meal, increase the meat, fish, or tofu portion.

Fat-Burning Dinner 6

SALMON BAKE

*Easy Oven Salmon

*Secret Yogurt Sauce

Grilled vegetables (zucchini, tomatoes, eggplant, bell peppers, fennel)

*Asian Slaw

Fat-Burning Dinner 7

COMFORT FOOD

*Hearty Meatloaf

*Mock Mashed Potatoes

Green beans

Fat-Burning Dinner 8

STEAK DINNER

6–8 ounces grilled skirt steak

Mixed grilled vegetables or *Sautéed Greens

Fat-Burning Dinner 9

TURKEY DINNER

6–8 ounces roasted turkey breast

1 pureed yam

Green beans

Fat-Burning Dinner 10

*DIJON AND PANKO-CRUSTED SALMON

Whole artichoke with lemon juice drizzle

*Salsa or Pico

*Baked Cinnamon Apple

Fat-Burning Dinner 11

PORTOBELLO-CHICKEN SUPPER

Large portobello mushroom grilled with tomato and onion

6–8 ounces roasted chicken breast

Steamed bok choy

Fat-Burning Dinner 12

SHRIMP DINNER

*Grilled Spicy Shrimp Salad

Cold asparagus spears dipped in 2 tablespoons *Secret Yogurt Sauce

*South of France–Style Chopped Salad

Fat-Burning Dinner 13

FAMILY-STYLE ROAST

*Crock Pot Roast

*Broiled Cauliflower

Green salad

Fat-Burning Dinner 14

BOUILLABAISSE

Mixed shellfish cooked in *Vegetable Stock with onion, garlic, saffron, and tomatoes

*Berrygood Yogurt

Fat-Burning Dinner 15

OLD-FASHIONED FAVORITE

*Chili-Avocado Chicken

*Mock Mashed Potatoes

*Sautéed Greens

Fat-Burning Dinner 16

BETTER THAN PASTA DINNER

*No-Noodle Lasagna

Mixed green salad with *Creamy Dressing

*Roasted Rapini

Fat-Burning Dinner 17

CURRY FAVORITE

*Coconut Curry Chicken

*Curry Cauliflower Soup

*Chocolate Yogurt

Tips for Dinner Success

- Never eat dinner when you are too hungry because you will eat grab-and-go foods and by the time your body registers that you have eaten them, it will be too late.

- Skip the steak sauces, which are loaded with sugar.

- Avoid added carbs for dinner. No added bread, beans, legumes, rice, potatoes, or chips for dinner. If you're still hungry, increase the portion sizes.

Red Flags

- Sauces tend to be loaded with flour and butter. This is not a good combination for your overall health or optimizing your Fat-Burning Machine.
- It is extremely easy to overeat salad dressings. Always put them on the side. If all you taste is salad dressing and not vegetables, you have a problem. Lemon juice and olive oil are always good alternatives to prepared dressings.

FAT-BURNING SNACKS

Be sure to eat three snacks a day to avoid getting overly hungry and to keep your Fat-Burning Machine working. In general, eat one snack midmorning, one snack midafternoon, and one snack in the evening. Here are some options:

- Cut vegetables (celery, carrots, bell peppers, sweet pea pods, cucumber, cauliflower, broccoli). Eat plain, or with a dollop of yogurt or blue cheese dressing.

- ½ cup *Guacamole, with cut veggies

- ¼ cup raw mixed almonds, walnuts, macadamia nuts, cashews, pecans

- Cold asparagus spears

- Celery sticks with 2 tablespoons peanut or almond butter

- 1–2 ounces whole or low-fat cheese

- Endive filled with cream cheese, tuna, or egg salad

- ½ avocado filled with cottage cheese

- Grilled peach or pear with cinnamon sprinkle

- Cauliflower florets with blue cheese dressing dip

- 1–3 ounces chicken, turkey, salmon, or tuna

- ½ cup plain 2% or whole-fat Greek yogurt

- 1 hard-boiled egg

- 2 *Deviled Eggs

- 1 cup chicken or vegetable broth

- ½ cup 2% or whole-fat cottage cheese (Can add artificial sweetener if needed. Cinnamon, vanilla, maple, or lemon extract can be used to taste.)

- One serving of fruit with any one of the following: 1 ounce deli meat, 1 ounce cheese, 1 tablespoon almond or sunflower butter, or ¼ cup 2% or whole-fat cottage cheese. Option is to add a few low-carbohydrate crackers and mustard. (Limit the fruit to occasionally, especially in the first couple of weeks, and don't snack on fruit if you've included it in a meal.)

- 1 apple and 8 ounces almond or soy milk

Tips for Snack Success

- Some people are sensitive to artificial sweeteners. Consumption of these products can cause insulin spikes. If you think you are sensitive, aim to significantly reduce or eliminate artificial sweeteners.

- Planning morning and afternoon snacks is important to help keep your Fat-Burning Machine ignited. These snacks can also prevent overeating in the evening. Plan to snack.

- Keep any after-dinner snacks sugar-free.

Red Flags

- Take one serving size of any snack and close the bag. Mindlessly overeating snacks directly from the bag is one of your biggest dangers. Avoid this pitfall by selecting one serving and closing the bag.

- Watch for hidden sugar in snacks that are nonfat. Prepackaged snacks are usually loaded with sugar.

DINING OUT

Being a Fat-Burning Machine means that you are in control of your eating and living life on your terms—not compromising or sacrificing. Eating out is an important part of your Fat-Burning Machine life. It is social, convenient, and tasty. There's no reason to be afraid of restaurants, as long as you know how to make good choices. Don't be shy about asking for substitutions or to have food prepared with sauces on the side.

Here are some guidelines that are helpful when you're dining out:

Tips for Restaurant Dining

- Check out the menu before you leave home. Many restaurants post their menus online. Make a note of the dishes that work for you so you won't get caught off-guard. Decide what you're going to eat ahead of time, and stick with your plan.

- Question everything on the menu. Just because it is a vegetable dish doesn't mean it is low in calories, and just because it is a meat dish doesn't mean it is high in calories. Some veggie dishes made with sauces, butter, and oils can have four times as many calories as some burgers that have only 250 calories.

- Start the meal with a salad of fresh greens that will ease your hunger.

- Move unlimited chips and bread away from you and toward someone else, or ask the server not to bring them. These are dangerous—
if you eat one, you'll likely eat the entire bowl. Be honest about the
potential for disaster. There is no reason to test your willpower.

- Restaurant sauces are often loaded with flour, sugar, and fat. This
is the worst combination of all foodstuffs. Also be extremely careful
with condiments. Sauces like honey mustard, barbecue sauce, and
ketchup are high in sugar, carbs, and calories. Know what you put
into your body.

- Fast-food restaurants aren't the best choice, but there are some
good options if you end up at these places. (See page 119.) Note
that many fast-food restaurants will wrap your burger in lettuce.
Skip the ketchup and barbecue sauces in favor of mustard and
mayo.

- Stay away from fried foods. Nothing good can come from eating
French fries, onion rings, tempura (even vegetable tempura), etc.

- Eat a small snack before you leave the house so you won't be ravenous.

- Order appetizer-size portions, or choose restaurants with a "small
plate" menu.

- Order an appetizer plus a salad for your main course, or share a
main course with a friend.

- If the restaurant serves large portions—for example, twelve ounces
of meat instead of eight—slice off the extra and set it aside for a
doggie bag.

- Regardless of the size of the entrée, stop eating when you're full.
Ask the waiter to wrap the leftovers to go.

- Avoid all-you-can-eat buffets.

- Skip dessert. It's a huge sugar hit at the end of a meal, and it's impossible to control the ingredients.

- Drink sensibly. Fruit juice, soda, sweet tea, and lemonade are all loaded with sugar and will trigger insulin and make you hungrier. Stick with water or unsweetened tea and coffee. (If you like a glass of wine with dinner, check the guidelines on page 82.)

Below is a guide for what to eat at some of the most popular restaurants—even fast food.

Chinese

Most Chinese restaurants have a healthy menu selection. Start there.

- Hot and sour soup

- Egg drop soup

- Whole steamed fish

- Tofu with vegetables (Sauce on the side. Similar to dressings, dip your fork or chopsticks in these toppings to control portion size.)

- Chicken with broccoli (Sauce on the side. Similar to dressings, dip your fork or chopsticks in these toppings to control portion size.)

- Broccoli or green beans with garlic

- Chow mein (meat or vegetable)

- Steamed entrées and vegetables (sauce on the side)

- Szechuan prawns

- Mu shu filling without wrappers

- Black bean sauce (on the side)

- Hot mustard

- Soy sauce

- *Carb options: ½ cup rice or 1 mu shu wrapper*

Japanese

- Miso or hot-and-sour soup
- Green salad with sesame dressing on the side
- Seaweed salad with dressing on the side
- Sashimi
- Negimaki
- Grilled meat or fish with teriyaki sauce on the side
- Grilled squid
- Asian barbecue
- Wasabi
- Fresh ginger
- *Carb options: ½ cup rice, ½ cup (shelled) edamame, or 1 small maki roll*

Korean

- Kimchi
- Steamed eggs
- Sweet potato noodles
- Bean sprouts
- Vegetable dishes—spinach, mushrooms, zucchini, greens
- Korean barbecue (beef, pork, or chicken cooked at the table)
- Pan-fried fish
- Clams with soybean paste
- Hot pot with meat, tofu, and vegetables

Mexican

- Fajita salad with chicken, shrimp, or beef (Ask for the salad on a plate and skip the deep-fried tortilla shell)

- Bean-less chili

- Small toppings of cheese, sour cream, and dressing on the side (Dip your fork in dressing)

- Grilled seafood, beef, or chicken with salsa on the side

- Guacamole

- Salsa (Unlimited salsa is OK)

- *Carb options: 1 small corn tortilla, ½ flour tortilla, or ½ cup black or pinto beans (not refried)*

Italian

- Salad with dark leafy greens, olive oil, and fresh garlic

- Caesar salad, easy on the croutons

- Caprese salad (mozzarella, tomato, and basil with olive oil)

- Antipasto (Cured meats, cheese, mushrooms, olives, artichoke hearts, pepperoncini)

- Italian egg drop or wedding soup (without pasta)

- Steamed clams or mussels

- Calamari salad

- Grilled or roasted vegetables

- Zucchini pasta (or other veggie-based "pastas," if available)

- Grilled or baked meat or fish with sauce on the side

Greek

- Greek salad with feta cheese and olives

- Grilled chicken or shrimp shish kebab with veggies

- Grilled lamb chops

- Chicken or lamb souvlaki

- Grilled vegetables

- Baba ghanoush

- Tzatziki sauce

- Tahini

- *Carb options: rice, small pita, 2 stuffed grape leaves, or 2–3 table-spoons hummus*

Indian

- Beef, chicken, or shrimp kebabs

- Meat or vegetable curries

- Roasted eggplant

- Chicken shorba soup (curried chicken and rice)

- *Carb option: ½ cup rice*

Barbecue

- Open-face sandwich or meat only. Pork, beef, or chicken are all good choices. Ask for the barbecue sauce on the side. Very, very small amounts of extra barbecue sauce—or none at all.

- Coleslaw

- Collard greens

- *Carb options: ½ cup black or pinto beans or ½ cup rice*

Seafood

- Lobster salad
- Fresh lobster
- Crab salad
- Fresh crab
- Fresh crayfish
- Calamari salad
- Steamed clams
- Raw oysters or clams
- Baked, sautéed, or grilled fish
- Coleslaw
- All seafood that isn't fried
- *Carb options: ½ bun on a lobster roll or ½ cup rice*

Mike's Fast-Food Guide

I treat fast-food restaurants as I do all other restaurants, with the same do's and don'ts. Just because food is "fast" doesn't mean that it has to be off my plan. It just means that I have to be exceptionally careful. Why? Because when I go to fast-food restaurants, I am the most at risk to sabotage my nutrition. The bites, licks, and tastes come into play, and I am tempted to "reward" myself for a job well done on becoming a Fat-Burning Machine. Or I just need to eat something quickly and might let my guard down.

Since I know that I am at risk in those situations, I have actually developed meal choices at most fast-food restaurants so that I can enjoy the food without sabotaging my progress.

Note that there are some sandwich choices on this list. Breakfast and lunch sandwiches every day—no matter how healthy the ingredients—will give you problems. But if you're traveling or stuck without other options, an occasional healthy sandwich is allowed.

Subway

My "go-to" fast-food restaurant is Subway. No matter where I am in the world, Subway is consistent, high-quality, fresh food. I love the fact that they prepare in front of me and I can choose specifically which bread, meats, vegetables, and condiments to include, as well as the quantities. Any sandwich can be ordered as a salad, and Subway posts the calorie count on their menu. Subway's Fresh Fit menu is full of healthy options.

My favorite sandwich is the six-inch turkey breast sub on nine-grain wheat bread. I usually get it toasted and add lettuce, tomato, green peppers, and spicy mustard. It can also be eaten as an open-face sandwich with only one slice of bread.

Starbucks

Starbucks is a very healthy option for us Fat-Burning Machines, but it can also be quite tempting. On the drink side, we all know to stay away from sweet drinks or "loaded" coffees. Hot or iced coffee is always good. Marcela loves the soy Tazo chai tea latte.

I find that the food at Starbucks is quite healthy. The chicken and black bean salad bowl, flatbread paninis, and wraps are reasonable choices. For lunch, I occasionally eat the roasted vegetable panini. It has zucchini, eggplant, peppers, sun-dried tomatoes, and baby spinach. Also as an occasional choice for breakfast, Starbucks has an amazing wheat wrap filled with cage-free egg whites, spinach, feta cheese, and tomatoes.

McDonald's

What makes McDonald's so great is that the restaurants are everywhere. What makes McDonald's a nightmare is that its menu is full of BLTs—the bites, licks, and tastes—(McNuggets, French fries, milk shakes) that will set me back. When I need to go to McDonald's, it is absolutely critical to know what I am going to eat and not let myself be tempted.

My favorite food at McDonald's—again, an occasional choice—is the Artisan Grilled Chicken Sandwich with lettuce, tomato, and no mayonnaise. I also eat only about half of the roll. This is a good option because it is a white-meat breast and is quite filling.

McDonald's also has amazing salads. The Premium Southwest Salad with Grilled Chicken and Premium Bacon Ranch Salad with Grilled Chicken are both great choices. The Ranch Snack Wrap also works well. Be very careful with the dressing. The best option is to use only oil and vinegar. If that is not an option, then use only about half the packet provided.

Stay away from Fruit 'N Yogurt Parfait and McCafé Strawberry Banana Smoothie. These are menu items that look healthy, but they are not. Too many carbs. It makes me hungrier than when I started.

For breakfast, McDonald's now offers an Egg McMuffin made with egg whites. It is made from 100 percent egg whites, extra-lean Canadian bacon, and white cheddar on an English muffin made with eight grams of whole grains. Not to eat every day, but it definitely works in a pinch.

Dunkin Donuts

Dunkin Donuts has a twenty-four-hour breakfast menu, which means you can get a healthy egg white sandwich all day. The turkey sausage or veggie egg white omelet with a slice of reduced-fat cheddar cheese, served on a multigrain flatbread, is also a good option.

Chipotle

I love Chipotle. Fresh ingredients, lots of choices, and local produce. There are many choices that work well for me. I like the freedom to design my food and have it made-to-order. The Burrito Bowl with black beans, fajita vegetables, lettuce, and chicken is amazing. I tend to stay away from guacamole, sour cream, and cheese because they add unnecessary calories and fat, but if you like them, use very small quantities on the side.

Taco Bell

Like McDonald's, Taco Bell is ubiquitous in its number of locations, but also its tempting BLTs. There is nothing to be gained by having a few nachos or a bite of a quesadilla. They'll turn off my Fat-Burning Machine.

Taco Bell's "Fresco Menu" has many good choices, including the Fresco Burrito Supreme with Chicken. Another good option is the chicken soft taco. (In both cases, you can eat the insides and not finish the entire wrapper.) A final option is the Cantina Bowl with its citrus-herb marinated chicken, black beans, guacamole, fresh pico de gallo, and roasted corn and pepper salsa, all served on a bed of premium rice. I'm careful to limit the dressing and only eat half of the rice.

Wendy's

Wendy was a healthy food pioneer. There are many choices that work well for me. The Asian Cashew Chicken Salad with Light Spicy Asian chili vinaigrette. The salad is topped with fire-roasted edamame, spicy roasted cashews, and warm grilled chicken. The Ultimate Chicken Grill Sandwich, an occasional choice, is layered with grilled chicken breast, honey mustard, lettuce, tomato, and onion.

Some other restaurant choices I like:

Chick-fil-A: Char-Grilled Chicken Garden Salad with Honey-Roasted Sunflower Kernels & Light Italian Dressing.

Pret À Manger: Wild Salmon Salad, featuring cucumbers, tomatoes, greens, tzatziki sauce, and lemon.

Panera: Half Smoked Turkey on Artisan Whole Grain Loaf plus Low-Fat Garden Vegetable Soup with Pesto or Mediterranean Chicken & Quinoa Salad.

Boston Market: The roasted turkey breast meal, paired with a side of fresh steamed vegetables.

Kentucky Fried Chicken: Grilled chicken breast dinner, complete with the spice mixture that made KFC famous. The chicken tastes great and has no carbs.

Fazoli's: Grilled Chicken Artichoke Salad with Lemon Basil Vinaigrette.

30-DAY QUICK MEAL PLAN

The following chart is a quick and easy way to help you plan meals for the first thirty days of your program. These are just suggestions. Go ahead and swap out meals for restaurant choices or leftovers. Switch a recipe (indicated in bold with an asterisk) with a simple meal of meat, fish, or tofu cooked as you like it. When quantities are not given—such as for vegetables—you can have an unlimited amount. For green salads, use either a simple oil-and-vinegar dressing (One tablespoon oil, one to two tablespoons vinegar) or choose from a dressing recipe in Chapter Nine.

30 DAY QUICK MEAL PLAN

	BREAKFAST	SNACK	LUNCH	SNACK	DINNER	SNACK
1	2 eggs scrambled with 1 oz cheese, tomato, and onion in 1 tbsp olive oil	¼ cup mixed raw nuts	*Turkey Blueberry Salad, vegetable or chicken broth	Cut veggies with ½ cup Greek yogurt	6–8 oz baked chicken, mixed green salad, *Broiled Cauliflower	1 serving sugar-free Jell-O or ice pop
2	*Salmon Breakfast Soufflé	½ cup Greek yogurt topped with shaved almonds	Spinach salad with hard-boiled egg, crumbled goat cheese, and 4–6 oz chicken	½ cup *Guacamole with cut veggies	*Zucchini Pasta, *Asparagus Soup Puree	Cucumber slices with 3 tbsp blue cheese dip or hummus
3	4–6 oz baked cod and veggies sautéed in 1 tbsp olive oil, ½ cup cottage cheese	¼ cup roasted chickpeas or pumpkin seeds	*Cauliflower Soup, mixed green salad	1 apple, 1 oz cheese	6–8 oz grilled or baked fish (any), steamed broccoli, *Asian Slaw	*Peanut Butter Oat Balls
4	1 cup Greek yogurt with high-fiber cereal and ¼ cup mixed berries	4–6 cold cooked asparagus spears dipped in 2 tbsp sour cream	*Grilled Spicy Shrimp Salad	2 slices tomato topped with 1–2 oz mozzarella and whole basil leaves	*Coconut Curry Chicken, ½ baked yam, mixed green salad	½ cup cottage cheese sprinkled with cinnamon

	BREAKFAST	SNACK	LUNCH	SNACK	DINNER	SNACK
5	2 eggs scrambled with veggies, 1 slice whole-wheat toast with 1 tbsp butter	Baby carrots, 2 tbsp hummus	2 lettuce and deli wraps with 1 slice each of deli turkey, ham, cheese	8 oz soy or almond milk, ¼ cup berries	Asian stir-fry with 6–8 oz beef, chicken, or shrimp and mixed vegetables in 2 tbsp olive oil, ½ cup rice	½ cup Greek yogurt
6	2 pan-fried eggs in 1 tbsp olive oil with 1 slice deli ham or sausage	2 flax crackers with 1 oz string cheese	*Poblano Pepper and Vegetable Chicken Soup, mixed green salad	Celery sticks with 2 tbsp peanut or almond butter	6–8 oz grilled or broiled skirt steak, grilled or oven-baked veggies	Sugar-free Jell-O or ice pop
7	*Steve's Easy Egg White Soufflé, ½ cup rice or quinoa	½ avocado, ½ cup cottage cheese	½ turkey sandwich on whole-wheat bread, 1 cup chicken or vegetable soup	5 olives with 1 oz cheese and 1 artichoke heart	*Easy Oven Salmon *Roasted Brussels Sprouts	Baby carrots, 2 tbsp hummus
8	2 pan-fried sausages cooked with kale in 1 tbsp olive oil, 1 slice whole-wheat toast or ½ English muffin	Endive leaves with 2 tbsp cream cheese and unlimited salsa	*Curry Cauliflower Soup, mixed green salad	¼ cup roasted pumpkin seeds	6–8 oz roasted turkey breast, ½ baked yam, green beans	*Chocolate Yogurt

	BREAKFAST	SNACK	LUNCH	SNACK	DINNER	SNACK
9	1 cup high-fiber cereal, 6 oz soy or cow milk, ½ cup cottage cheese	Celery and cherry tomatoes with 2 tbsp blue cheese dip, 1 hard-boiled egg	*Seafood Stew, mixed green salad	1–2 oz cheese with a handful of raw nuts	*No-Noodle Lasagna, steamed broccoli, mixed green salad	1 serving sugar-free Jell-O or ice pop
10	2 poached eggs, 1 sliced tomato, 1 slice whole-wheat toast	Celery sticks with 2 tbsp peanut or almond butter	*Gale's Health Salad, choice of soup or ½ *Creamy Chicken Salad sandwich	2 tbsp hummus with cut veggies	*Hearty Meatloaf, *Mock Mashed Potatoes, green beans	*Peanut Butter Oat Balls
11	½ cup oatmeal, 6 oz milk or soy milk, ½ cup mixed berries	1 oz hard cheese, 1 piece beef or turkey jerky	*Smoked Salmon Salad or Wrap	3 stuffed grape leaves	*Balsamic-Dijon Chicken or any roasted chicken, *Roasted Rapini	¼ cup baba ghanoush with cut veggies
12	*Athlete's Omelet	½ cup Greek yogurt	BLT salad, ¼ cup cantaloupe slices	¼ cup raw mixed nuts	*Chicken Pesto Chimichurri over Sautéed Spinach	Sugar-free Jell-O or ice pop

	BREAKFAST	SNACK	LUNCH	SNACK	DINNER	SNACK
13	1 cup high-fiber cereal, ½ cup Greek yogurt, 2 tbsp shaved almonds	1–3 oz sliced deli turkey or ham	*Roasted Eggplant with Raw Vegan Pesto	¼ cup sesame seeds	Pan-fried catfish (or any fish), *Asian Slaw, steamed kale	¼ cup mixed raw nuts or sesame seeds
14	*Salmon Breakfast Soufflé	¼ cup roasted chickpeas, 1 pepperoni stick or 1 piece beef or turkey jerky	*South of France–Style Chopped Salad	4 mushroom caps stuffed with 2 tbsp cream cheese	*Crock Pot Roast, roasted zucchini or sweet peppers	½ cup *Guacamole with cut veggies
15	*Omelet Burrito	2 flax crackers with 1 oz cheese	*Salmon Cilantro Salad, 1 slice whole-wheat bread	¼ cup baba ghanoush with cut veggies	Asian stir-fry with chicken, beef, or shrimp, ½ cup rice	1 rice cake with 1–2 tbsp peanut or almond butter
16	½ cup oatmeal, 6 oz cow or soy milk, 5 oz tomato juice	½ cup Greek yogurt	*Ratatouille, 1 tin sardines with 3 flax crackers	1 cup chicken or vegetable broth	6–8 oz baked cod (or any fish), grilled veggies	Sugar-free Jell-O or ice pop

	BREAKFAST	SNACK	LUNCH	SNACK	DINNER	SNACK
17	*Take-and-Go Egg Cups	¼ cup mixed raw nuts	*Slow Cooker Texican Chili, mixed green salad	5 olives with 1 oz cheese and 1 artichoke heart	*Chili-Avocado Chicken, *Mock Mashed Potatoes, *Sautéed Greens	1 rice cake with 1–2 tbsp peanut or almond butter
18	1 cup high-fiber cereal, 6 oz rice or soy milk, 5 oz vegetable juice	1 apple, 1 oz hard cheese	1 baked chicken thigh, *Asian Slaw	1 cup *Asparagus Soup Puree	6–8 oz grilled or baked tilapia (or any fish), steamed artichoke with lemon juice, mixed green salad	3 stuffed grape leaves
19	*Asparagus and Goat Cheese Frittata	½ cup roasted pumpkin seeds	*Curry Cauliflower Soup, ½ cup rice	2 *Deviled Eggs	6–8 oz roasted chicken or turkey, steamed or grilled vegetables	*Berrygood Yogurt

	BREAKFAST	SNACK	LUNCH	SNACK	DINNER	SNACK
20	2 egg whites cooked with mixed vegetables in 1 tbsp olive oil, 1 slice whole-wheat toast with 1 tbsp butter	¼ cup mixed nuts	*Creamy Chicken Salad, lettuce, tomato	½ cup *Guacamole with cut veggies	*Chicken Esquites, steamed baby bok choy	1 pear, 1 oz hard cheese
21	1 cup Greek yogurt with 1 cup high-fiber cereal, 6 oz tomato juice	1 apple sliced and spread with 1 oz cream cheese	2 cooked 4-oz hamburger patties with tomato, lettuce, onion, and mustard	1 rice cake with 1–2 tbsp peanut or almond butter	*Easy Oven Salmon *Roasted Brussels Sprouts	*Chocolate Yogurt
22	*Athlete's Omelet	¼ cup mixed raw nuts	*BLT Wrap	1 cooked artichoke sprinkled with lemon juice	6–8 oz baked or grilled fish (any), steamed or grilled veggies	*Baked Cinnamon Apple
23	*Salmon Breakfast Soufflé	¼ cup baba ghanoush with cut veggies	3 oz canned tuna with 1 tbsp mayo on 1 slice whole-wheat bread	¼ cup roasted pumpkin seeds	6–8 oz pork chops, steamed or grilled veggies	½ cup mixed berries, 6 oz rice or soy milk

	BREAKFAST	SNACK	LUNCH	SNACK	DINNER	SNACK
24	½ cup oatmeal, 6 oz cow or soy milk, ¼ cup mixed berries	2 flax crackers with 1 oz cheese	*Omelet Burrito	½ avocado, 1 chopped tomato and chopped scallions with oil and vinegar drizzle	6–8 oz roasted turkey breast, ½ baked yam, green beans	*Berrygood Yogurt
25	2 eggs scrambled with 1 oz cheese, tomato and onion in 1 tbsp olive oil	¼ cup roasted chickpeas	*Slow Cooker Texican Chili, mixed green salad	½ cup Greek yogurt, cut veggies	6–8 oz baked chicken, steamed asparagus, mixed green salad	1 grilled pear with cinnamon sprinkle
26	1 cup Greek yogurt, 1 cup high-fiber cereal, ¼ cup mixed berries	½ avocado with ½ cup cottage cheese	½ turkey sandwich, 1 cup vegetable soup	2 flax crackers with 1 oz string cheese	*Hearty Meatloaf, *Mock Mashed Potatoes, green beans	*Peanut Butter Oat Balls
27	2 pan-fried sausages cooked with kale in 1 tbsp olive oil, 1 slice whole-wheat toast or ½ English muffin	2 *Deviled Eggs	*Salmon Cilantro Salad, ½ cup quinoa	2 strips turkey jerky	*Chili-Avocado Chicken, grilled veggies	½ cup Greek yogurt

	BREAKFAST	SNACK	LUNCH	SNACK	DINNER	SNACK
28	2 eggs scrambled with veggies in 1 tbsp olive oil, 1 slice whole-wheat toast with 1 tbsp butter	¼ cup almonds, 2 raw carrots	Spinach salad with hard-boiled egg, crumbled goat cheese, and 4–6 oz chicken	½ cup Greek yogurt, cut veggies	*Slow Cooker Beef and Vegetable Chili, mixed green salad	*Peanut Butter Oat Balls
29	1 cup Greek yogurt with 1 cup high-fiber cereal, 6 oz tomato juice	¼ cup mixed raw nuts	*Turkey Blueberry Salad, 1 cup *Asparagus Soup Puree	2 pepperoni sticks or 2 pieces beef or turkey jerky	6–8 oz grilled or broiled lamb chops, green salad with feta cheese and olives, grilled veggies, tzatziki sauce	Sugar-free Jell-O or ice pop
30	Egg white omelet with 1 oz cheese and veggies of choice cooked in 1 tbsp olive oil, 1 slice whole-wheat toast with 1 tbsp butter	Celery sticks with 2 tbsp peanut or almond butter	Asian stir-fry with chicken, beef, shrimp, or tofu cooked in 2 tbsp olive oil, ½ cup rice	¼ cup roasted pumpkin seeds	*Easy Oven Salmon, *Roasted Rapini	½ cup Greek yogurt, ¼ cup mixed berries

As you can see from these menu plans, restaurant and fast-food options, and 30-Day Quick Meal Plan, this diet isn't about punishing yourself. It's about retraining your palate and making the best fat-burning decisions. There are a wide variety of choices. If you're like me, you'll discover that you love eating this way and no longer crave the foods that were making you overweight and unhealthy. That's the big bonus of the Fat-Burning Machine Diet.

NINE

OUR FAVORITE FAT-BURNING RECIPES

Loving the food you eat is the most important part of becoming a Fat-Burning Machine. Having food that is easy to make, doesn't take a ton of time, and can be purchased in any store is also important. Gale and her team of Fat-Burning Machine chefs (Danielle Polansky, Delbert Bernhardt, Linda Kennedy, Samantha Tritsch, Steve Gilbert, and Scott Ellis) created these wonderful recipes that are delicious, practical, and best of all, fat burning. If you don't have a grill for the grilled recipes, you can bake, broil, or pan-fry the meat or fish instead.

Enjoy!

SALADS

TURKEY BLUEBERRY SALAD

4 cups chopped spinach

6 ounces turkey breast (roasted or deli)

½ cup fresh blueberries

¼ cup chopped pecans

2 tablespoons olive oil

2 teaspoons balsamic vinegar

On a plate of spinach, layer chopped turkey, blueberries, and pecans. Drizzle olive oil and balsamic vinegar over the top as dressing.

Serves 1

Danielle Polansky

SALMON CILANTRO SALAD

1 pound cooked salmon fillet, cooled

¼ cup diced scallion

¼ cup diced celery

2 tablespoons minced cilantro

2 tablespoons balsamic vinegar

2 tablespoons olive oil

Salt and pepper to taste

Slice the salmon into bite-size chunks, removing the skin and bones. Place the pieces in a medium mixing bowl. Add remaining ingredients and mix well. Chill and serve.

Serves 2-3

C. Whitney

CREAMY CHICKEN SALAD

2 cups diced cooked boneless, skinless chicken breast

⅓ cup Greek yogurt

⅓ cup mayonnaise

¼ cup diced celery

¼ cup diced onion

Salt and pepper to taste

Mix all ingredients together, chill, and serve.

Serves 4

C. Whitney

GRILLED SPICY SHRIMP SALAD

*Spicy Fish Marinade (page 172; full recipe, reserving 1 tablespoon)

1 pound medium or large shrimp, shelled and cleaned

¼ cup red onion, sliced in thin rings

1 onion, sliced in thin rings

1 green bell pepper, sliced

3 cups romaine, chopped

1 tablespoon *Secret Yogurt Sauce (page 173)

1 tablespoon *Guacamole (page 174)

Make Spicy Fish Marinade and let shrimp marinate in the mixture in a large covered bowl for at least 30 minutes.

Use the reserved tablespoon of Spicy Fish Marinade and sauté onion and green bell pepper.

Grill shrimp 3 minutes each side.

To assemble salad: On a bed of romaine, place onion, bell pepper, and red onion. Top with grilled shrimp and dress with Secret Yogurt Sauce and Guacamole.

Serves 2–3

Danielle Polansky

ASIAN SLAW

1½ cups shredded red cabbage

1½ cups shredded green cabbage

1 cup grated or julienned carrot

3 scallions, sliced thin

½ cup chopped cilantro, leaves only

1 cup sliced bok choy

1 red bell pepper, diced

1 yellow bell pepper, diced

1 tablespoon black sesame seeds

2 tablespoons tamari

3 tablespoons rice vinegar

3 tablespoons sesame oil

1 inch fresh ginger, grated

Dressing:

Shred cabbage as thin as you can. (I use a mandoline.) Place cabbage in a bowl and add the carrots, sliced scallions, cilantro, bok choy, red bell pepper, yellow bell pepper, and black sesame seeds.

Whisk the dressing in a small bowl and pour over salad.

Serves 2-3

Danielle Polansky

SOUTH OF FRANCE–STYLE CHOPPED SALAD

2 heads romaine

1 head radicchio

1 red bell pepper

1 orange bell pepper

A mixture of yellow and red cherry or grape tomatoes

3 baby cucumbers

One avocado, cut into bite-size squares

1 jar hearts of palm, drained and cut into bite-size circles

½ can plain chickpeas

Homemade dressing:

½ cup olive oil

Juice from 1 fresh lemon (discard the seeds)

1–2 tablespoons Dijon mustard, to taste

1 teaspoon raw honey

Handful chopped fresh basil

1 teaspoon oregano

Salt and pepper to taste

To make the dressing: In a small mixing bowl, pour in the olive oil. Squeeze in the lemon juice. Add Dijon mustard and mix through. Once the mustard starts to break up, add raw honey and continue mixing. Throw in the chopped fresh basil, the teaspoon of oregano, salt, and freshly ground pepper; all spices can be modified to taste. Continue to mix really well with a whisk or spoon, or put in a container so you can shake it up. You can serve immediately with salad, or refrigerate and save for another time. This stays fresh for a full week.

For the salad, finely cut or chop the romaine, cutting from the top down to the bottom in very thin amounts, to get a fully chopped texture. Place in a large serving bowl. Then cut the radicchio in the same way and place in the bowl with the romaine. Cut up the peppers into small bite-size squares, and add to the lettuces. Cut up the yellow and red baby tomatoes, and put into the salad. Slice the baby cucumbers, each piece into fours, and add to the salad. Add the avocado and hearts of palm. Drain the chickpeas and add on top. Once you have all the ingredients in the salad, mix until they are combined. Mix in dressing and serve.

Serves 4–6

Samantha Tritsch

GALE'S HEALTH SALAD

2 cups greens (mixed greens, spinach, or kale)

½ yellow bell pepper, cut into dime-size pieces

½ cup cauliflower, cut into dime-size pieces

½ cup sweet pea pods, cut into dime-size pieces

½ cup cherry or Cherub tomatoes (yellow are my preference), cut in half

½–1 cup carrot slices, cut into dime-size pieces

½–1 cup English cucumber, cut into dime-size pieces

1 tablespoon olive oil

1–2 tablespoons balsamic vinegar or flavored vinegar (cherry, raspberry, or peach)

Place the greens into a large mixing bowl. Using kitchen scissors, chop the greens into bite-size pieces. (It is easiest to do this by putting one hand on each side of the scissors and using them in a vertical position, randomly going around the bowl chopping.)

Put all remaining ingredients into the bowl and toss. Eat immediately, or allow salad to rest in the refrigerator while preparing other items.

As a main meal with protein, salad will make 1–2 servings.
As a side salad, it will make 3–6 servings.

Gale Bernhardt

SOUPS AND CHILI

VEGETABLE STOCK

1 leek

1 onion

1 tablespoon olive oil

1 clove garlic

6 cups water

2 carrots

2 stalks celery

3 shiitake mushrooms

2 sprigs fresh parsley or
1 teaspoon dried

2 sprigs fresh thyme or
½ teaspoon dried

1 bay leaf

1 teaspoon salt

1 tablespoon black peppercorns

Slice onion and leek, and sauté them in olive oil in a skillet until onion begins to turn translucent. Add garlic and cook 2 more minutes until fragrant. Place water, onion, leek, garlic, carrots, celery, mushrooms, parsley, thyme, bay leaf, and salt in a stockpot and cook on low for a minimum of 1½ hours. You may also throw this in a Crock-Pot (increase water by 2 cups) and cook on low all day.

This will be a base for many soups. This stock will last in the fridge for 1 week or up to 3 months in the freezer.

Danielle Polansky

CAULIFLOWER SOUP

1 onion, chopped

2 cloves garlic, chopped

1 tablespoon olive oil

6 cups water

1 medium-size cauliflower

1 teaspoon sea salt

2 tablespoons nutritional yeast (found in grocery baking section)

In stockpot, sauté chopped onion and garlic in olive oil. Cook until onion becomes translucent. Add water and quartered cauliflower. Cook on medium heat for 20–30 minutes or until cauliflower is soft. Pour ingredients into high-power blender and blend. Add salt and nutritional yeast. Chill. Garnish with sliced scallions.

Serves 2–3

Danielle Polansky

CURRY CAULIFLOWER SOUP

1 onion

2 cloves garlic

1 head cauliflower

1–2 tablespoons curry powder (more or less to your taste)

16 ounces chicken broth

½ teaspoon salt

1 can (13.5 ounces) full-fat coconut milk

1 teaspoon olive oil

Fresh parsley or basil to garnish

Finely chop the onion and garlic. In a large pot, cook the onion and garlic in olive oil until the onion is translucent. Chop the cauliflower into small pieces. Put in the pot and sprinkle curry powder over cauliflower until coated. Add the chicken broth and salt. Cover with a lid and cook the cauliflower until very tender. Add the can of coconut milk and heat on low until heated through, stirring frequently. Remove from heat. Blend the soup in a blender until a creamy consistency. Garnish each bowl of soup with chopped parsley or basil.

Serves 4

Linda Kennedy

ASPARAGUS SOUP PUREE

1½ pounds asparagus

4 tablespoons ghee (clarified butter) or butter

1 cup chopped onion

4 cloves garlic, minced

2 cups thinly sliced carrots

2 cans (14.5 ounces each) low-sodium chicken broth

½ cup minced fresh parsley

2 tablespoons minced fresh basil

1 tablespoon minced fresh cilantro

Salt and pepper to taste

Cut the tips off of the asparagus and set them aside. Cut the remaining stalks into 1-inch pieces. In a saucepan, melt the butter and then sauté the onion and garlic until both are tender. Add the carrots and asparagus pieces and cook for roughly 3 minutes. Then stir in the chicken broth, parsley, basil, and cilantro. Cover and simmer the mixture until the vegetables are tender—about 3 to 6 minutes.

Allow the mixture to cool slightly before pureeing the soup in a food processor or blender. Return the mixture to the pan, adding the asparagus tips. Cook long enough to make the asparagus tips tender.

Serves 4-6

Delbert Bernhardt

ASIAN SOUP WITH BAKED TOFU

1 package firm tofu

3 tablespoons olive oil

2 tablespoons tamari or soy sauce

1 tablespoon fish sauce

½ teaspoon grated fresh ginger

6 cups vegetable stock

2 heads baby bok choy

3 carrots

1 cup bean sprouts

2 scallions

½ red bell pepper

1 small zucchini

1 cucumber

¼ cup cilantro

1 lime

1 jalapeño

Sriracha paste

Strain off the liquid from the tofu. Pat the tofu dry with a paper towel. In a separate small bowl, combine olive oil, tamari or soy sauce, fish sauce, and fresh ginger. Baste both sides of the tofu with the mixture using a basting brush. Bake at 400°F for 20 minutes on each side.

Chop all the following and add into warm stock right before you eat: bok choy, shredded carrots, bean sprouts, scallions, red bell pepper, shredded zucchini, cucumber, baked tofu, cilantro, lime, jalapeño, and sriracha paste. (The jalapeño and sriracha paste are to add heat.)

The baked tofu is good to have already prepared in fridge.

Serves 4

Danielle Polansky

POBLANO PEPPER AND VEGETABLE CHICKEN SOUP

1 whole chicken

3 cups water

4 medium poblano peppers, seeded and diced

32 ounces low-sodium chicken stock

½ –1 pound baby carrots

1 pound sliced mushrooms

1 bag (1 pound) frozen peas

1 bag (1 pound) frozen green beans or 3–4 cups fresh green beans

1 zucchini, sliced

1 yellow squash, sliced

1 red bell pepper, seeded and sliced

1 orange bell pepper, seeded and sliced

2 bay leaves

Onion powder and garlic powder to taste

In a very large, deep pot, boil the chicken until a drumstick pulls free, about 60 to 90 minutes. Remove the chicken from the pot and add all remaining ingredients. While vegetables are cooking, remove the chicken meat from the bone and add it back to the pot. Simmer until vegetables are still firm and chewy. This freezes well.

Serves 4

Gale Bernhard

SLOW COOKER TEXICAN CHILI

1½ pounds top sirloin steak, cut into ½-inch cubes

2 cans (1 large 28-ounce can and 1 small 14.5-ounce can) stewed
   tomatoes

2 cans (8 ounces each) unsweetened tomato sauce

1 cup sliced carrots

1 medium onion, chopped

1 cup chopped celery

1 cup chopped green bell pepper

1 tablespoon chopped garlic

1 tablespoon ancho chili powder (or chopped ancho chili)

¼ cup minced fresh parsley

1 teaspoon salt

½ teaspoon ground cumin

¼ teaspoon black pepper

Brown the beef in a skillet. Then transfer it to a 5-quart slow cooker.
Add all remaining ingredients. Cover and cook on low heat for 9 to 10
hours, stirring occasionally. This freezes well.

Serves 16–18

Delbert Bernhardt

SLOW COOKER BEEF AND VEGETABLE CHILI

1½ pounds lean ground beef

1 can (14.5 ounces) stewed tomatoes with onion, celery, and bell pepper

1 can (10 ounces) tomato juice

1 cup chopped celery

1 cup chopped yellow or green bell pepper

½ cup chopped carrots

1 teaspoon salt

1 teaspoon pepper

1 tablespoon garlic

3 tablespoons chili power

2 teaspoons ground cumin

OPTIONAL: 1 can (15 ounces) dark red kidney beans, rinsed and drained

Brown ground beef and drain. Rinse and drain kidney beans, if using.
Mix all ingredients in a slow cooker. Cover and cook on low for 6 hours.
Serve with sour cream, scallions, and cilantro, if desired.

Serves 4

Delbert Bernhardt

POBLANO WHITE CHILI

1 pound ground turkey

2 tablespoons olive oil

1 cup diced celery

1½ cups fresh, diced poblano peppers

½ small can (4.5 ounces) hot diced green chilies

1 cup chopped sweet onion

4 cups low-sodium chicken broth

2 cups seeded and diced fresh tomatoes (roughly 4 Roma tomatoes)

2 cups seeded and diced fresh zucchini (roughly 2 small)

½ teaspoon salt

½ teaspoon ground cumin

⅛ teaspoon cayenne pepper

Black pepper to taste

Brown the ground turkey in the oil in a medium saucepan. Drain excess drippings. Add celery, poblano peppers, chilies, and onion to the meat and cook until tender.

Add all remaining ingredients and blend well. Bring the mixture to a boil, reduce the heat, and simmer for 30 minutes or until flavors are well blended. Serve in bowls.

Just prior to serving, add toppings, such as: fresh, diced jalapeno peppers, diced avocado, chopped cilantro, diced tomato, and shredded cheddar cheese (if you use avocado, eliminate the cheese).

Serves 4

Gale Bernhardt

MAIN COURSES

CHICKEN ESQUITES

2 chicken breasts

1 tablespoon olive oil

Juice of 1 lemon

Salt and pepper

2 cups cottage cheese

Zest and juice of ½ lime

Dash cayenne pepper

2 cups chopped spinach

2 cups chopped tomatoes (any variety)

3 scallions, chopped

1 red bell pepper, chopped

1 cup chopped cilantro

3 radishes, chopped

Marinate chicken in olive oil, lemon juice, and salt and pepper to taste. Grill or bake chicken at 375°F until fully cooked through.

Mix cottage cheese, lime zest and juice, and cayenne pepper. Set aside. Chop chicken into small cubes.

Layer in a jar: spinach, tomato, cottage cheese mixture, scallions, chicken, red bell pepper, cilantro, and radishes.

This will store for up to 3 days in the refrigerator. It's a great to-go option for lunch.

Serves 2

Danielle Polansky

ZUCCHINI PASTA WITH ROASTED TOMATOES & CHIMICHURRI

2 medium-size zucchini

½ onion

1 clove garlic

1 tomato

3 tablespoons *Chimichurri (page 174)

Sea salt and pepper to taste

Shred zucchini into threads. You can use a cheese grater, julienne slicer, or mandoline. Set aside.

Thinly slice the onion. Mince the garlic. Sauté the onion in 1 tablespoon chimichurri. Add the zucchini and sauté for 2–3 minutes. The key is to not overcook the zucchini (think al dente).

Slice the tomato and place on foil in a broiling pan. Sprinkle with sea salt and pepper. Bake at 400°F for 15–20 minutes or until edges are brown.

Create a bed of zucchini, place a few tomatoes on top, and pour 2 tablespoons chimichurri sauce over the top.

Serve with grilled or baked chicken.

Serves 4

Danielle Polansky

CHICKEN PESTO CHIMICHURRI OVER SAUTÉED SPINACH

2 chicken breasts

Salt and pepper to taste

½ onion

1 tablespoon olive oil

4 cups spinach

2 tablespoons tamari or soy sauce

1–2 tablespoons *Chimichurri (page 174)

2 tablespoons chèvre

¼ cup milk

¼ cup pine nuts

Season chicken breasts with salt and pepper. Grill for 6 minutes each side.

Slice onion and sauté in olive oil in a saucepan. Add spinach and pour tamari over greens. Cook on medium heat just until spinach wilts.

In a separate saucepan, place chèvre and milk on low heat and whisk until incorporated.

Toast pine nuts in oven at 300°F for about 8 minutes.

Serve grilled chicken over greens and drizzle chèvre and chimichurri over the top. Sprinkle with pine nuts.

Serves 2

Danielle Polansky

HEARTY MEATLOAF

2 eggs

3 pounds lean ground beef

1 cup chopped onion

¼ cup chopped red bell pepper

¼ cup chopped green bell pepper

¼ cup chopped garlic

¼ cup sour cream

¼ cup fresh horseradish

¼ cup chili sauce

2 teaspoons oregano

½ cup grated cheddar cheese

Preheat oven to 350°F. Mix eggs and beef first. Then mix in the remaining ingredients until blended well. Form the mixture into a loaf and place in an olive oil–wiped baking dish. Cover and bake for 70 minutes. Uncover and bake an additional 10 minutes or until internal temperature is at 155°F.

Serves 9

Delbert Bernhardt

NO-NOODLE LASAGNA

3 medium or 4 small zucchini

1 pound ground turkey sausage, ground beef, or Italian sausage

1 red onion, chopped

2 jars (14 ounces each) no-sugar-added spaghetti sauce

2 cups ricotta cheese

2 eggs

½ cup Parmesan cheese

1 tablespoon chopped fresh parsley

3–4 cups shredded Italian blend or mozzarella cheese

Cut zucchini into thin slices lengthwise to mimic lasagna noodles. If you have a vegetable slicer or mandoline, it makes the slices a uniform thickness. Set aside.

Brown meat and break up into small pieces. Add chopped onion and cook until onion is translucent. Add 1 jar of spaghetti sauce to meat and set aside.

In a separate bowl, mix ricotta, eggs, Parmesan, and parsley; set aside.

To the bottom of a large pan, spread ⅓ jar of spaghetti sauce.

Layer zucchini over sauce, slightly overlapping the slices.

Add ½ of the meat mixture and spread over zucchini.

Pour ⅓ jar of spaghetti sauce over meat.

Spread ½ of ricotta mixture over meat layer and spread evenly.

Spread ½ of Italian/mozzarella cheese on top.

Finish a second layer the same as the first (zucchini, meat, sauce, ricotta, shredded cheese).

Bake at 350°F, placing the pan on a cookie sheet to catch any cheese for 60–75 minutes. Check at 45 minutes and cover with foil if cheese is getting too brown.

Serves 4

Linda Kennedy

COCONUT CURRY CHICKEN

2 tablespoons curry powder

1 tablespoon coconut palm sugar

½ teaspoon paprika

½ teaspoon coriander

1 teaspoon oregano

½ teaspoon salt

2 tablespoons coconut oil

2 large chicken breasts, cut into 1-inch pieces

1 onion, chopped

2 cloves garlic, minced

1–2 red bell peppers, cut into 1-inch pieces

1 can (13.5 ounces) full-fat coconut milk

In a small bowl, combine curry powder, coconut sugar, paprika, coriander, oregano, and salt. Set aside.

In a large skillet, melt coconut oil. On high heat, brown the chicken on both sides. Chicken will not be cooked through yet. Remove from pan.

Lower heat to medium. Add onion and garlic to the pan and cook until onion is translucent.

Add red peppers and browned chicken. Sprinkle spice mix over chicken and stir until spices cover the chicken and vegetables and become fragrant.

Turn heat to low. Add the can of coconut milk. Cook for 10–15 minutes, stirring frequently until chicken is cooked through.

Serve over wilted kale or spinach.

Serves 2

Linda Kennedy

CHILI-AVOCADO CHICKEN

4 medium to large green chili peppers (mild to spicy—your choice—
  examples: poblano, jalapeño, hatch green)

4 chicken breasts

Salt and pepper

Garlic powder

1 teaspoon olive oil

4 slices provolone cheese

2 avocados, sliced

Lime juice

Roast chilies in a skillet, turning them until skin is blistered all over. When skin is charred, put in a bowl and cover with foil to steam the chilis. When cool enough to touch, remove the skin, cut in half, and remove the seeds.

Sprinkle chicken with salt, pepper, and garlic powder. Drizzle with olive oil and grill until fully cooked through.

Top each grilled chicken breast with roasted chile and 1 slice provolone cheese. Return to the grill to melt the cheese. Top with avocado slices and fresh lime juice.

Serves 4

Linda Kennedy

SEAFOOD STEW

1 tablespoon olive oil

1 medium onion, diced

½ cup diced red bell pepper

1 tablespoon crushed garlic

1 can (14.5 ounces) diced tomatoes, undrained

1 can (10.75 ounces) condensed tomato soup

2 cups hot water

1 can (8 ounces) tomato sauce

½ teaspoon dried basil

½ teaspoon dried oregano

1 teaspoon dried parsley

1 tablespoon Worcestershire sauce

1 jar (2 ounces) pimentos, undrained

1 teaspoon red pepper flakes

Salt and pepper to taste

1 bag (16 ounces) frozen bay scallops

1 can (6.5 ounces) crab (in fresh seafood refrigerated area)

2 cans (10 ounces each) whole baby clams

40 cooked cocktail shrimp, tails removed (thawed if using frozen)

In a Dutch oven, sauté olive oil, onion, red pepper, and crushed garlic until onion and pepper are soft. Add tomatoes, tomato soup, hot water, tomato sauce, basil, oregano, parsley, Worcestershire sauce, pimentos, red pepper flakes, salt, and pepper. Cook over medium heat for 15 minutes.

Add scallops, crab, and clams. Increase heat and bring to a boil. Add shrimp and simmer for an additional 10 minutes.

Serves 4

Delbert Bernhardt

CROCK-POT ROAST

1 (4.5–5-pound) cross-cut beef roast

Greek seasoning

4 poblano peppers

1 orange or red bell pepper

4 stalks celery

1 cup baby carrots

1 can (10 ounces) Ro-Tel diced tomatoes with habaneros

2 tablespoons crushed garlic

Onion powder to taste

Salt and pepper to taste

1 can (12 ounces) low-sodium beef broth

Rub roast generously with Greek seasoning. Slice and cut poblano peppers into ½-inch pieces. Slice and cut bell pepper into ½-inch pieces. Slice and cut celery stalks into ½-inch pieces. Slice carrots into ½-inch pieces (or leave whole). Drain diced tomatoes and habaneros. Mix all vegetables with garlic, onion powder, salt, and pepper in a large bowl.

Place roast in a 7-quart Crock-Pot. Add Beef broth. Place vegetable mix around roast to slightly cover. Set Crock-Pot on low and cook for 6 hours.

Serves 4–6

Delbert Bernhardt

BALSAMIC-DIJON CHICKEN

1 cup balsamic vinegar

2–3 tablespoons Dijon mustard

1 clove garlic, minced

Salt and pepper to taste

Fresh basil

4–6 pieces thinly sliced chicken breast

Coconut oil spray or other vegetable oil spray (to coat pan)

Make the balsamic mixture in a mixing bowl large enough to accommodate the chicken. Mix together balsamic vinegar and Dijon mustard. Add minced garlic and continue mixing. Add salt and pepper to taste. Continue mixing. Add the basil and mix. The basil will largely float back to the top of the mixture, but that is OK.

Bathe each piece of chicken in the balsamic mixture, being sure to cover both the bottom and top, and mix the chicken around (don't just drop them in!). After each has been covered with the balsamic mixture, leave the chicken in the bowl and refrigerate for at least 30 minutes, or overnight. (If you are making it on the fly, 30 minutes is fine. I try to refrigerate for at least an hour.)

Heat oven to 400°F on the roast setting, or 425°F on the bake setting.

Spray oil onto a baking sheet. Remove the chicken from the refrigerator and place each piece onto the sheet. With a spoon, dribble an additional spoonful of the balsamic mixture onto each piece of chicken, making sure to get at least 1 piece of basil on each. When ready, place the chicken into the oven. Let cook for 30–40 minutes, until it starts to crisp on the outside. At 30 minutes, check the chicken by cutting a tiny slice with a sharp knife and making sure it is cooked through. Serve immediately with any roasted vegetable, brown or wild rice, or with a salad.

Serves 4–6

Samantha Tritsch

DIJON AND PANKO-CRUSTED SALMON

Coconut oil spray (to coat pan)

1 pound salmon, cut into 2 portions

Salt and pepper to taste

Dijon mustard

1 cup panko bread crumbs (preferably whole-wheat)

Heat the oven to 400°F. While the oven heats up, spray a baking sheet or pan with coconut oil spray. Wash the salmon and pat dry, then place onto the baking sheet. Sprinkle a dash of salt and pepper on each piece. With a butter knife, coat a thin layer of the Dijon mustard on top of each piece of salmon. Sprinkle the panko bread crumbs on each piece, just a light, thin layer. Place the fish into the oven and bake for 15 minutes. If you prefer the salmon to have an extra crispy layer, broil for an additional 2–3 minutes. Serve immediately.

Serves 2

Samantha Tritsch

EASY OVEN SALMON

Olive oil

4–6 ounces salmon per person

Salt-free seasoning of choice (favorites include Greek and Cajun)

Move the top oven rack 2 positions away from the top broiling position. Turn the oven on broil.

Layer two pieces of aluminum foil and fold up all the edges to make a pan. Lightly brush the foil with olive oil. Place salmon on the foil and lightly brush the top of the salmon with olive oil and season to taste.

Cook 3–5 minutes, depending on salmon thickness and personal preferences. Move the rack to the top position and cook an additional 2–5 minutes.

Gale Bernhardt

VEGETABLES

SAUTÉED GREENS

1 onion, chopped

1 tablespoon olive oil

1 clove garlic, minced

4 cups greens (spinach, kale, collard greens, bok choy)

1–2 tablespoons tamari

Sauté onion and olive oil in skillet over medium heat until onion becomes translucent. Add garlic and cook for 1–2 minutes more. Turn up the heat and add greens and tamari and cook until they just begin to change color. Remove from heat immediately.

Serves 4

Danielle Polansky

ROASTED RAPINI

1 bunch rapini (also known as broccoli rabe), sliced evenly, not chopped, retaining stems

2 tablespoons olive oil

Salt and pepper

Place rapini on cookie sheet and drizzle olive oil over the top. Season with salt and pepper. Bake at 400°F for 20 minutes or until leaves are crunchy to the touch.

Serves 4

Danielle Polansky

BROILED CAULIFLOWER

1 head cauliflower

¼ teaspoon salt

Spices of choice:

Italian (Italian seasoning, Parmesan cheese)

Indian (curry, basil, turmeric)

Irish (dill, thyme)

Mexican (chili powder, paprika, oregano)

½ teaspoon olive oil

Slice cauliflower into thin slices. Place on cookie sheet. Sprinkle cauliflower with salt and your favorite combination of spices. Drizzle with olive oil. Broil or grill until edges are browned.

Serves 4

Linda Kennedy

RATATOUILLE

½ onion, chopped

1 tablespoon minced garlic

½ teaspoon olive oil

1 tablespoon Italian seasoning

2 cans (14.5 ounces each) stewed tomatoes

1 can (6 ounces) tomato paste

½ cup water

1 small eggplant, trimmed and very thinly sliced

1 zucchini, trimmed and very thinly sliced

1 yellow squash, trimmed and very thinly sliced

1 red bell pepper, sliced into thin rings

1 yellow bell pepper, sliced into thin rings

2 tablespoons olive oil

Salt and pepper to taste

1 tablespoon each fresh basil and thyme leaves, or to taste

OPTIONS

¾ pound turkey sausage, browned and crumbled

2 tablespoons crumbled goat cheese

In a saucepan, cook onion and garlic in ½ teaspoon olive oil until translucent. Add Italian seasoning and stir until fragrant. Add stewed tomatoes, tomato paste, and water. Cook on low for 10–15 minutes. Remove from heat and blend tomato sauce with immersion blender or in food processor until smooth.

Spread the tomato sauce on the bottom of a large casserole dish. Arrange alternating slices of eggplant, zucchini, yellow squash, red bell pepper, and yellow bell pepper on top of the sauce, slightly pressing the vegetables into the sauce. Overlap the slices a little to display the colors. Drizzle the vegetables with remaining 2 tablespoons olive oil and season with salt and pepper. Sprinkle with basil and thyme leaves. Cover vegetables with a piece of parchment paper cut to fit inside the pan. Cook at 375°F for 45 minutes. Remove the parchment paper for the last 15 minutes.

OPTIONS: Top vegetables with cooked sausage before putting in the oven. Serve with crumbled goat cheese.

FASTER OPTION: Use a jar of no-sugar spaghetti sauce instead of making the tomato sauce.

Serves 4–6

Linda Kennedy

ROASTED BRUSSELS SPROUTS

1 package fresh Brussels sprouts, or about 25 sprouts

2 tablespoons olive oil

Salt and pepper to taste

Wash Brussels sprouts and cut off ends and outer leaves. Cut in half and place on a cookie sheet. Drizzle olive oil over the top and season with salt and pepper.

Bake at 400°F for about 20 minutes, or until edges turn slightly golden in color.

Serves 4–6

Danielle Polansky

ROASTED EGGPLANT WITH RAW VEGAN PESTO

1 large eggplant, sliced ½-inch thick

Ingredients for raw vegan pesto:
½ cup olive oil
Juice of ½ lemon
Handful of basil (or to taste)
1–2 cloves garlic (or to taste)
¼ cup sprouted sunflower seeds
6–10 raw, unsalted cashews
1 teaspoon coarse sea salt
Handful of raw kale, de-stemmed
Coconut oil spray or any vegetable spray (to coat pan)

Make pesto by combining ingredients in a food processor or on the pulse setting of a blender for about 30 seconds. For a thinner consistency, add ½ cup water or additional extra-virgin olive oil to taste. Continue to blend until the consistency is to your liking. Set aside.

Turn the oven to 400°F on roast. Spray coconut oil (or any type of preferred oil cooking spray) onto a baking pan and place the eggplant on top. Sprinkle a dash of olive oil, coarse sea salt, and pepper on the eggplant pieces. Then, cover each slice of the eggplant with a thin layer of the pesto. Once you have covered each piece of eggplant, place the baking sheet into the oven. Roast the eggplant for 15–20 minutes, until crisp and golden brown in color. Remove from the oven and serve with additional pesto on the side. Pesto is good for a full week, so feel free to refrigerate the remainder and use throughout the week.

Serves 2

Samantha Tritsch

MOCK MASHED POTATOES

½ head cauliflower

½ cup water

½ teaspoon salt

2 tablespoons cream cheese

1 tablespoon Parmesan cheese

¼ teaspoon nutmeg

1–2 tablespoons milk (more or less as needed for desired consistency)

Chop cauliflower into small pieces. Put in a spaghetti pot with ½ cup water. Cover with a lid and cook the cauliflower until tender. Drain the water. Mash the cauliflower with the salt and cheeses in a food processor or with a potato masher. Add enough milk to create a similar consistency to mashed potatoes.

Serves 4

Linda Kennedy

EGGS

ATHLETE'S OMELET

1 teaspoon olive oil

1 large egg

2 egg whites

½ cup brown rice or quinoa (precooked and chilled)

¼ cup chopped tomatoes or Cherub tomatoes cut in half

½ cup chopped fresh spinach

¼ cup chopped sweet yellow, red, or orange bell pepper

Lightly coat the bottom of a small skillet with the olive oil. Stir the egg and egg whites together in a small bowl and set them aside. On medium heat, lightly cook the vegetables so they remain crispy. Add the egg mixture and the rice at the same time. Cook the mixture until the eggs are firm and moist, but not hard.

Serves 1

Gale Bernhardt

OMELET BURRITO

2 whole eggs or 1 egg plus ⅓ cup egg whites

1 tablespoon milk

¼ teaspoon salt

¼ teaspoon pepper

½ teaspoon butter

¼ avocado, mashed

¼ red bell pepper, cut into thin slices

Whisk eggs and milk and season with salt and pepper. Melt butter in an 8- to 10-inch skillet. Cook egg mixture on low to medium heat in a very thin layer to mimic a tortilla. Flip to cook on both sides. Remove to a plate and let cool slightly. Spread avocado on egg and add pepper slices. Carefully roll up like a tortilla and wrap in foil or waxed paper. This recipe is easy to take with you for breakfast or lunch on the go.

Serves 1

Linda Kennedy

TAKE-AND-GO EGG CUPS

12 foil cupcake liners

12 slices deli ham or turkey

1 cup egg whites

¼ teaspoon salt

¼ teaspoon pepper

OPTIONAL

¼ red bell pepper, finely chopped

¼ cup Italian-blend shredded cheese

Fill muffin pan with foil cupcake liners.

Place 1 slice of ham or turkey into each foil liner, folding it in carefully to be able to hold the egg whites. It will look like a flower petal.

Mix egg whites with salt and pepper. Pour roughly 2 tablespoons egg whites into each foil liner. Top each egg cup with optional red peppers and cheese.

Bake at 350°F for 20–25 minutes.

Serves 4–6

Linda Kennedy

STEVE'S EASY EGG WHITE SOUFFLÉ

Olive oil to coat

1 cup sliced mushrooms

½ cup fresh chopped green beans

¾–1 cup Egg Beaters

Wipe a soufflé dish with olive oil. Put the mushrooms and beans in the bottom of the dish. Cover with Egg Beaters. Microwave for 8 minutes on high.

Serves 1

Steve Gilbert

DEVILED EGGS

6 eggs, boiled, cooled, and peeled

1½ tablespoons light or regular mayonnaise

1 tablespoon Dijon mustard

¼ cup chopped dill pickle

Paprika to sprinkle

Cut eggs in half, lengthwise. Scoop out the yolks and place them in a small bowl. Mash the yolks and mix with mayonnaise, mustard, and pickle, creating a smooth consistency. Place egg halves on a plate, and spoon mixture into each of them. Chill and serve. Top with a sprinkling of paprika.

Serves 3

C. Whitney

ASPARAGUS AND GOAT CHEESE FRITTATA

4 tablespoons olive oil

¼ onion, finely chopped

4 spears asparagus, chopped into 1-inch pieces

1 small red bell pepper, chopped

1 teaspoon Italian seasoning

¼ teaspoon crushed red pepper flakes

10 large eggs

3 tablespoons milk (or 2% Greek yogurt)

¼ teaspoon salt

¼ teaspoon ground black pepper

¼ cup grated Gruyère cheese

4 ounces soft goat cheese, crumbled

2 tablespoons chopped flat-leaf parsley

Preheat broiler. Heat 1 tablespoon olive oil in large ovenproof nonstick skillet over medium heat. Add the onion, asparagus, red bell pepper, Italian seasoning, and red pepper flakes. Cook, stirring occasionally, until the vegetables are soft—about 7 minutes. Transfer to a small bowl and cool; don't wash the skillet.

Beat the eggs, milk (or yogurt), salt, and pepper in a large bowl. Stir in the cooked vegetables. Heat the remaining 3 tablespoons olive oil in the nonstick skillet over medium heat. Pour in the egg mixture and spread the vegetables evenly throughout the pan. As the eggs set, lift the edges to allow the liquid eggs to run underneath. Cook until the eggs are mostly set but the center is still a little runny—10–15 minutes.

Sprinkle the Gruyère and goat cheese over the top and broil until the top is golden brown—about 2 minutes. Remove the skillet from broiler and loosen the edges of the frittata. Cool for 10 minutes in the skillet. Slide frittata onto a serving platter, slice, and serve.

Serves 4

Scott Ellis

SALMON BREAKFAST SOUFFLÉS

1 tablespoon diced shallot

½ red bell pepper, chopped

½ cup shredded kale

2 eggs

4 egg whites

3 tablespoons milk

¼ cup feta cheese

½ cup smoked salmon

2 tablespoons thinly sliced red onion

2 tablespoons capers

1 tablespoon olive oil

6 parchment baking cups

Sauté onion, shallot, and red bell pepper. Add kale and sauté until just cooked. Mix eggs, egg whites, and milk. In a large bowl, whisk egg mixture, feta, sautéed vegetables, smoked salmon, red onion, and capers. Pour into parchment baking cups. (This is key, since regular baking cups will stick.) Bake at 350°F for 20 minutes or until a toothpick inserted in the center comes out clean.

Serves 2–3

Danielle Polansky

SANDWICHES, WRAPS

Sandwiches are not a regular part of the Fat-Burning Machine Diet. But they're allowed every two weeks or so as a treat. Avoid them altogether in the first two weeks of the diet.

DANIELLE'S SUPER SANDWICH

4 ounces deli-sliced or fresh-baked turkey breast

1 tomato, chopped

1 teaspoon olive oil

⅛ teaspoon garlic salt

1 slice whole-grain bread, toasted

¼ avocado

1 tablespoon *Secret Yogurt Sauce (page 173)

Handful of sprouts for topping

Sauté turkey breast and ½ chopped tomato in olive oil in a saucepan. Add garlic salt. Turkey will slightly brown on the edges. Spread avocado on toast. Pour Secret Yogurt Sauce on top of avocado. Slice the other half of the tomato. Place sautéed turkey over avocado and then top with tomato and sprouts.

This can also be served over a bed of lettuce using the Secret Yogurt Sauce as the dressing and cutting up the avocado.

Serves 1

Danielle Polansky

SMOKED SALMON SALAD OR WRAP

Prepare as either a salad or a wrap.

Romaine leaves (about 3)

1 red onion, sliced

4 ounces smoked salmon slices

1 cucumber, sliced thin

1 teaspoon capers

1 lemon, juiced

1 low-carb sandwich wrap

1 tablespoon whipped cream
cheese

Salad:

On a bed of romaine, place sliced red onion, smoked salmon, and cucumber. Sprinkle capers and lemon juice over the top. Omit cream cheese and wrap.

Wrap:

On a low-carb wrap, spread whipped cream cheese. Place chopped romaine, red onion, salmon, cucumber, and capers on top. Squeeze lemon juice over the top and fold into a wrap.

Serves 1

Danielle Polansky

BLT WRAP

1 tablespoon mayonnaise or ranch dressing

1 low-carb tortilla wrap

½ cup shredded lettuce

1 small tomato, chopped

2–3 slices cooked bacon

Spread a thin layer of mayonnaise or ranch dressing on the wrap. Add shredded lettuce, then chopped tomato. Cut bacon slices in half and add on top of lettuce and tomato. Fold into a wrap.

Serves 1

DESSERTS

Desserts are a challenge on the Fat-Burning Machine Diet. That's because sugar and even artificial sweeteners used in some "sugar-free" recipes are not optimal for fat burning. This handful of dessert recipes should be reserved for special occasions and avoided altogether during the first two weeks of the diet.

PEANUT BUTTER OAT BALLS

2 cups whole oats

1 scoop protein powder

1 teaspoon chia seeds (optional)

1 cup creamy nut butter (no-sugar-added peanut, almond, or cashew)

½ cup coconut palm sugar

¼ cup water

2 tablespoons cocoa powder

2 tablespoons cinnamon

½ teaspoon salt

1–2 tablespoons unsweetened shredded coconut (optional)

Mix oats, protein powder, and chia seeds in a large bowl. In a microwave-safe dish, add all other ingredients except the coconut. Heat on low or defrost setting until the nut butter becomes pliable and you can mix the ingredients together. Add the wet ingredients to the oat mixture and stir with a spoon (or your hands) until the mixture is combined. Add 1 teaspoon of water at a time if you need more liquid to make the oats combine with the "dough." Use a cookie scoop to create approximately 40 small balls. If you like coconut, pulse the shredded coconut into small pieces in a food processor. Roll the balls in the coconut. Store in the refrigerator.

Serves 15–20

Linda Kennedy

CHOCOLATE YOGURT

1 cup Greek yogurt

1 teaspoon unsweetened cocoa powder

½ teaspoon cinnamon

2–5 drops of vanilla extract or maple flavoring

OPTIONAL: 1 packet artificial sweetener

Mix all ingredients together. An option is to use ½ cup Greek yogurt and ½ cup low-fat cottage cheese for a heartier-tasting dessert.

Serves 1

Gale Bernhardt

BERRYGOOD YOGURT

½ cup ripe raspberries

½ cup ripe blueberries

1 cup Greek yogurt

Puree ¼ cup each of raspberries and blueberries in a food processor or blender.

Remove and stir the puree into the yogurt. Top with remaining whole berries.

Options: Substitute strawberries or blackberries for raspberries or blueberries.

Use ½ cup yogurt and ½ cup cottage cheese.

Serves 2

Gale Bernhardt

BAKED CINNAMON APPLE

Parchment paper

2 large Jonathan or Fuji apples, cored

2 tablespoons ground cinnamon

Preheat oven to 400°F. Line a baking sheet with parchment paper. Wash and cut each apple into 6–8 slices. Place on the parchment-covered baking sheet and sprinkle with cinnamon. Bake for 10 minutes, then turn over and sprinkle the other side with cinnamon. Continue baking for 10 minutes.

Serves 2

C. Whitney

SAUCES/DRESSINGS

CREAMY DRESSING

4 tablespoons olive oil

2 tablespoons fresh lemon juice

½ teaspoon Dijon mustard

1 tablespoon feta cheese

½ tomato, chopped

1 teaspoon sea salt

4 leaves fresh basil

1 tablespoon chopped shallot

Place all ingredients in a blender or food processor and puree.

Danielle Polansky

SPICY FISH MARINADE

¼ cup olive oil

½ teaspoon sea salt

½ teaspoon cayenne pepper

¼ cup lemon juice

1–2 cloves garlic, minced

1 teaspoon cumin

¼ cup chopped fresh cilantro

Mix all ingredients in a bowl. Great as a marinade for fish, vegetables, shrimp, and chicken.

Danielle Polansky

SECRET YOGURT SAUCE

1 container (17 ounces) 2% Greek yogurt
¼ cup *Salsa or Pico

Mix yogurt with salsa and use as a salad dressing or sauce on sandwiches.

Danielle Polansky

SALSA or PICO

3 medium tomatoes
1 jalapeño, seeds discarded
½ teaspoon sea salt
¼ teaspoon black pepper
¼ onion, minced
¼ cup chopped cilantro
Juice of ½ lime

Place all ingredients except onion and cilantro in blender. Pulse until blended. Don't leave on blend or it will become frothy. After incorporated, stir in onion and cilantro.

PICO: Use the same ingredients, but slice tomatoes, jalapeno, and onion very small. Stir in remaining ingredients.

Danielle Polansky

CHIMICHURRI

1 cup flat-leaf parsley

1 cup cilantro leaves

1 clove garlic, minced

½ cup olive oil

1 tablespoon apple cider vinegar

½ teaspoon sea salt

Place all ingredients in a food processor or high-powered blender and blend until smooth.

Danielle Polansky

GUACAMOLE

1 ripe avocado

Juice of ½ lime

¼ teaspoon sea salt

Dash black pepper

1 tablespoon chopped cilantro

¼ orange bell pepper, chopped

2 tablespoons minced red onion

Mash avocado. Add lime juice, salt, pepper, cilantro, bell pepper, and red onion.

Serves 2

Danielle Polansky

BEST-EVER TOMATO SAUCE

2 cloves garlic, minced

Extra-virgin olive oil

2 cans (28 ounces each) whole peeled tomatoes

Fresh basil, torn and chopped

1 teaspoon coarse sea salt

Kosher sea salt

Freshly ground black pepper

1–2 tablespoons roasted red pepper flakes (optional)

Set a large cooking pot over medium heat. Add the minced garlic with a dash of olive oil and cover until brown, about 1 to 2 minutes. Meanwhile, remove all the whole tomatoes from the cans into a blender, discarding any additional sauce. Pulse the tomatoes together, about 45 seconds, until desired consistency. If you prefer more of a smooth puree, pulse for just over a minute. Once the garlic has browned, uncover the pot, turn heat down to a high simmer (be careful with the hot garlic and oil, as it tends to pop), and add in the tomato mixture. Then, add in the chopped basil. Mix and add two large dashes of olive oil, continuing to stir. Add in coarse sea salt and a generous dash of kosher salt and black pepper. Mix until all ingredients are combined. Cover and let simmer for at least 40 minutes. Taste the sauce as it simmers, every 20 minutes or so, and add any combination of olive oil, kosher salt, or pepper to taste. For those who enjoy a spicy kick, add red pepper flakes to the sauce. Once done, you can serve immediately or jar and refrigerate for weeks. If you freeze the sauce, it can last for months!

Serves 6–8

Samantha Tritsch

LOW-SUGAR BBQ SAUCE

2 cups low-sugar ketchup

¼ cup coconut palm sugar

2 tablespoons apple cider vinegar

1 tablespoon Worcestershire sauce

1 teaspoon balsamic glaze

¼ teaspoon allspice

¼ teaspoon cinnamon

Mix all ingredients in a saucepan and cook over low heat for 5–10 minutes, stirring frequently. Freeze leftovers.

Linda Kennedy

——

TEN

STRATEGIES TO GET MOVING

An Introduction to Fat-Burning Workouts

I am definitely a morning person. I have no problem waking up early and getting to work. As I said before, I don't really like gyms. I prefer to do as much of my aerobic exercise outside as I can. I like running or biking in the morning when I am fresh.

Nothing is more glorious to me than an early morning run in Central Park with my iPod, listening to my favorite tunes and getting my thoughts together for the day. The cool air, the hustle and bustle of the morning commuters, and the smell of the city energize me. I love to people-watch. Since I travel a lot, I also like to use my runs to sight-see. I will circle famous parks, see historical sites, and run on the banks of the great rivers of the world. Running in Hyde Park in London, around the Pearl Necklace in Mumbai, the Champs-Élysées in Paris, or the boardwalk in Santa Monica energizes me and makes me want to do more.

So I start most of my mornings with a run or a bike ride on an empty stomach. I alternate days between Miracle Intervals and endurance to keep my Fat-Burning Machine strong. And I've learned an important lesson that I want to impart to you: If you incorporate exercise into your life and do the things you love to do, it will become synonymous with pleasure—not just a grim routine you *have* to do.

> If you incorporate exercise into your life and do the things you love to do, it will become synonymous with pleasure—not just a grim routine you *have* to do.

Gale and I designed this plan so that you can jump into any of the exercise programs at the level that suits you best. The workouts in the next chapter are tailored to different fitness levels. Begin by finding the fitness level that describes you best. If you find that none of the levels match your personal situation, select the lowest level that most clearly matches yours. It's always possible to add more training intensity to a plan.

MEASURING EXERCISE INTENSITY

To gauge exercise intensity, we will use what scientists call ratings of perceived exertion, or RPE. In short, your level of exercise is described by how you feel. As you advance in your endurance exercise adventures, other tools such as heart rate monitors, pace, and power meters (exercise intensity on a bicycle shown in watts) can be used. Even if you use these additional tools, it's still important to gauge how you feel.

Here are the levels:

FAT-BURNING EFFORT 1 (FBE1): This is a very easy, steady, rhythmic pace. Your breathing is gentle, yet above your non-exercise breathing rate.

FAT-BURNING EFFORT 2 (FBE2): Breathing rate and exercise pace increases slightly. Breathing is a little deeper, but still comfortable. Your sweat rate is more than FBE1, but holding a conversation is possible. You can sing the "Happy Birthday" song while doing this effort.

FAT-BURNING EFFORT 3 (FBE3): Breathing increases in tempo and depth. Conversation becomes more broken. You could sing the "Happy

Birthday" song, but not without pauses in the wrong spots of the song in order to catch your breath. This zone can be considered the tempo zone for those familiar with training with devices such as heart rate monitors.

FAT-BURNING EFFORT 4 (FBE4): Your breathing becomes hard; the pace is fast. If you were to sustain this pace for more than about two minutes, singing and conversation would come out in two- or three-word segments with plenty of breathing between the words. For those who are currently fit, this is the highest effort you could sustain for about an hour going at your current all-out-fast pace. This zone can be considered the lactate threshold zone for those familiar with training with devices such as heart rate monitors.

FAT-BURNING EFFORT 5 (FBE5): This is maximum effort for durations of three minutes or less. There is a wide range of speeds here. For those who are fit, an all-out 20-second effort is a sprint. An all-out three-minute effort is not a sprint, but is significantly faster than FBE4.

WHAT TO DO ON DAYS OFF

You will notice that every plan has scheduled days off. Depending on your personal fitness and lifestyle needs, you may need to take these days to tend to other obligations. In any of the plans, you can add a steady walk of 20 to 45 minutes on your day off if you have the time and energy. Many people find that a lunchtime walk helps them feel energized for the rest of the day. Eat lunch before or after the walk.

Watch what you eat. This is a danger day because exercise actually helps suppress your appetite. If you decide you don't feel like taking a walk on your day off, then find something else constructive or relaxing to do with your time. Research new recipes; treat yourself to a massage; look for strength-training exercises that are a variation of those shown in the book; read up on high-value, nutrient-rich foods; meditate; or do anything other than floating around the kitchen like a shark looking for something to bite.

MAKING IT WORK

When you look at each plan, notice that workouts are shown on particular days. For example, strength training might be shown on Tuesday and Thursday. If it works better for you to strength-train on Monday and Wednesday, it's OK to move things around within a week. Be flexible, but have resolve. If you plan a workout for later in the week, be sure you can fit it in.

Be careful not to stack all of the workouts on the weekend. Things get busy for everyone. If you end up skipping all of your midweek workouts, rather than having an exercise binge on the weekend, just repeat that week of the plan again. No reason to freak out; just be patient. You didn't get here in a week, and it will take longer than a week to get you out of it.

Be sure you have decent footwear for your sport. That is, don't use your fancy office shoes for fast walking, jogging, or running. Go get the right footwear for your sport. Have fun with it.

Do not—seriously—do not make every workout session as difficult as possible. It will just make you not want to do it. Exercise has to be associated with pleasure. The old phrase "no pain, no gain" does not apply to you. It's not that some workouts shouldn't be tough, or that parts of some workouts are uncomfortable. Discomfort helps you stretch and achieve new levels of fitness. Flogging yourself through every exercise session leads to mediocre workouts, injury, and overtraining. This is counterproductive to your goals of fat burning. Use the intensity guidelines in your plan to help you succeed. Remember that the whole point of fitness is to make you feel more alive. The workouts should give you energy and a sense of well-being.

MIRACLE INTERVALS

You will find short intervals with long recovery periods in every plan. In the early plans, the intervals—typically some 10 to 30 seconds long—are accelerations. To accelerate means to build speed throughout the time shown on the plan. These accelerations help to train your nerves and muscles to move more quickly.

After you've built some fitness in nerves, tendons, ligaments, and muscles, you can add more speed, beginning with the next zone of effort. If you have a higher level of fitness, you can sprint. (If you have a heart rate monitor, you'll need to ignore it for these intervals because they are too short to get a decent heart rate response.)

The overachievers reading the plan are surely thinking, "Bah! I don't need long recoveries at an easy pace. What a waste of time." Or maybe the thought is, "I can do much more than 30 seconds. I'm no wimp. I can do one or two minutes instead."

Don't succumb to this false logic. The Miracle Intervals are a core component of this program. Believe it or not, the *miracle* of Miracle Intervals comes from the recoveries, not the accelerations, so enjoy the "downtime." You earned it.

MORNING WORKOUTS ON AN EMPTY STOMACH

I like to do my workouts early because it is the best way to ensure that I actually do them. Also, I have the most control of my mornings and don't risk something coming up or someone needing something urgently. Finally, when I do my workouts in the morning, I can tell people about it all day.

I began to see better results when I started doing my morning workout on an empty stomach. This is something athletes know to do, but among amateurs there's a misconception that you need to eat first for energy. Instead, exercising with limited carbohydrate availability forces cells to produce energy via fat oxidation rather than using easy-to-access glucose from a recent meal. Burn the glucagon in the morning. You will also find that you are less hungry for breakfast.

A recent study looked at twenty young males participating in an endurance-training program that lasted six weeks. Before telling you about the test results, know that in this particular study, the subjects were on a high-carbohydrate diet. That said, half of the group performed their training in a fasted state, while the other half of the group consumed around 640 carbohydrate calories before the session and a high-carbohydrate drink during the session. The study yielded a couple of interesting results. First, it found that the fasting group *did not* develop an exercise-induced drop in blood glucose concentration—or low blood sugar. Second, researchers concluded that the fasting group was more effective than the carbohydrate-fed group at increasing the muscles' ability to burn fat, as well as increasing the muscles' ability to use oxygen.

Another study conducted back in 2010 found that training in a fasted state while consuming a daily diet that is rich in fat (50 percent fat) was more effective in improving glucose tolerance and insulin sensitivity—in other words, burning instead of storing fat. If you track calories and macronutrients, you will find that the diet recommended in this book will put your fat calories around that 50 percent mark.

To clarify, don't get the impression that all workouts need to be done in the morning on an empty stomach. They do not. Also, do not get the impression that all exercise should be done on only water and no supplemental calories—that is not the case. Here's a general rule of thumb:

WORKOUTS LESS THAN 60 MINUTES: You don't need a snack before your workout. Nor do you need to consume a sugary sports drink during your workout. The supplemental calories are not necessary for this duration. In particular, there is no place for sugary sports drinks in your diet. Drinking them outside of very specific situations will not make you better at your sport; it will only make you fat.

LOW-INTENSITY EXERCISE SESSIONS: No matter the duration, these sessions do not require "energy" or sports drinks. Just eat regular meals and snacks during the workout or sport session as if it were a nonexercise session. Examples include a walk or easy hike. If your hiking intensity is FBE2 and above for extended periods of time, follow guidelines in the next two sections.

WORKOUTS LESS THAN 90 MINUTES AT FBE1 OR FBE2: During the workout, use water only. Within 60 minutes after this workout, eat your normal fat-burner breakfast.

WORKOUTS 90 TO 120 MINUTES LONG AT LOW INTENSITY: If the workout is 90 to 120 minutes long, begin on an empty stomach. At intensity FBE1 and FBE2, either no additional calories are needed or some athletes will need to fuel a small amount beginning around 60 or 90 minutes. For these athletes, consume about 50 to 75 calories of a chewy sports product made of tapioca solids or syrup and water. Natural tapioca syrup supplies glucose that gets absorbed into our bloodstream immediately, and it also contains complex carbohydrates that digest more slowly, taking two or three hours. Of course the slow-digesting solids won't help if you eat one at the 90-minute mark and you quit exercising at 120 minutes, but they shouldn't spike your insulin response.

Another option is to have a bite of a sports bar that is roughly 40–55 percent carbohydrate. If you use a bar or eat some real food like part of a peanut butter sandwich, be sure to chew it well and wash it down with water. (Be chill with the sports bar. A bite is a bite. If you eat the whole bar because it is there or it tasted good or some other reason, you will defeat the purpose.)

WORKOUTS 90 TO 120 MINUTES LONG AT HIGH INTENSITY: For 90- to 120-minute, high-intensity workouts (FBE3–FBE5), you can do a couple of things. For 90-minute workouts you can do two eating bouts split any way you please, consuming a total of 50–100 calories. After the workout, consume your normal fat-burner breakfast. For workouts that are 120 minutes, there are two choices:

1. Consume 50 calories at each 30-minute mark, including the end of the workout. This means roughly 50 calories at 30, 60, 90, and 120 minutes.

2. Skip the last feeding at 120 minutes. In all cases, consume a normal breakfast within 60 minutes of finish.

VERY LONG WORKOUTS EXCEEDING 120 MINUTES: If you are an athlete coming to this program and you are already doing long workouts, know that adapting to the diet will take three weeks or so. If you jump right into the fueling guidelines below, you may not feel so great during your workouts. Just know that is likely to happen. If this is the case for you, you will likely need to design your own hybrid system that is some of what you used to do and some of what we recommend here.

Because you're going to be out for a long time, there are a couple of options. First, you can begin on an empty stomach like you have in shorter workouts. The second option is to eat your normal breakfast and then begin your long workout after one or two hours.

If you begin on an empty stomach, you can then begin fueling your workout as described in the section "Workouts 90 to 120 Minutes Long at High Intensity." Be certain you are hydrating to thirst, somewhere around 22 ounces per hour.

STAYING HYDRATED

If your workout will include FBE3 and higher sustained intensities, carry one bottle of sports drink with electrolytes and one bottle of water. Preferably, your sports drink should contain sodium citrate rather than sodium chloride.

Sodium citrate is better than sodium chloride (table salt) because exercise stress causes blood to be shunted away from digestion and toward working muscles. Blood is also shunted to the surface of the skin to aid in body cooling. Often, a second layer of stress is added by exercising in hot and/or humid environmental conditions. These stresses change fluid regulation in the body.

The key to any hydration process is fast absorption of water and electrolytes in the intestinal cells. In a resting condition, chloride is a key ion in this absorption process. But during exercise, immune and inflammation reactions occur due to reduced blood flow to the gut. These reactions change the membrane potential of the cells and stimulate the release of chloride ions. The release of chloride ions sets off a series of reactions, ultimately leading to gut cramping and diarrhea.

With sodium citrate, the citrate ion can be used as part of what is known as the citric acid (or Krebs) cycle of energy production. This cycle involves chemical reactions that generate energy. Because citrate is metabolized differently than chloride during exercise, gastrointestinal problems are eliminated.

Similar to the recommendations in the section for Workouts 90 to 120 Minutes Long at High Intensity, fuel at a rate of around 100 to 150 calories per hour. The count begins after the first 30 minutes. Some athletes are able to go as low as 50 calories per hour, while others find they need more than 150 calories per hour. You will need to experiment to see what works best for you.

HOME STRENGTH-TRAINING FAT-BURNING EXERCISES

Strength is a key to fat burning, so strength training plays a role in this program.

You will find the strength exercises beginning in Phase II of Level I—charted in the next chapter. There are four categories of strength exercises: hip extensions, chest presses or push-ups, abdominal exercises, and back extensions. The instructions for each exercise are detailed below. If you're a beginner, do only enough repetitions so you are in control of the movement. For some people, this will be 3 sets of 3–5 repetitions. For others it will be 3 sets of 10–12 repetitions. As you progress through the training plan, you can aim for 3 sets of 15–20 repetitions.

Hip Extension Exercises

a. Chair Sit

Choose a stable chair for this exercise. Just as you might imagine, turn away from it and slowly sit down in the chair. Use a foot and leg position that feels natural for you. Your goal is to use your leg muscles to control the lowering motion into the chair. Hold your arms loosely at your sides. Do not allow yourself to plop into the chair as you sit by releasing all leg muscles and control. Once in the chair, pause for 1 to 2 seconds and then, again using your legs, stand up. Concentrate on your leg muscles as you stand. If you are just beginning, you may want to position the chair next to a table so you can use the table as balance and support by putting one hand on the table to help you up and down. As you gain strength and balance, you can slowly minimize and then eliminate using the table for support. Another tip for beginners is to use a chair that is set higher or has a pillow or two in it, graduating to a lower chair as you gain strength. Complete 12 to 15 repetitions or as specified on your training plan.

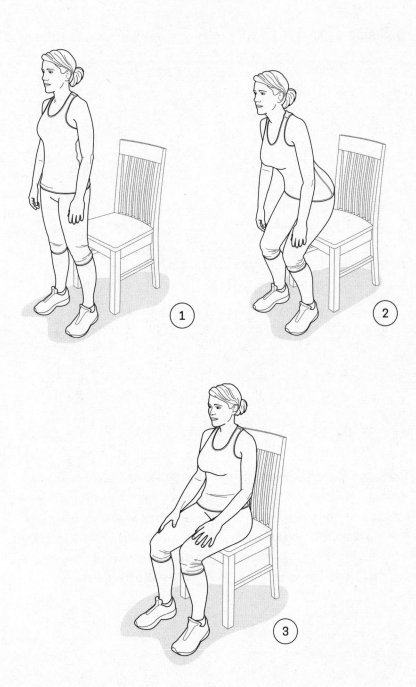

b. Squat

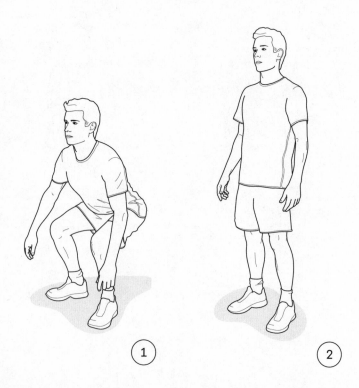

1

2

The Squat is the same movement as the Chair Sit, except there is no longer a chair used. Your movements down and up are slow, smooth, and controlled—legs managing all of the weight—with no rest taken between squatting down and standing back up. One option is to stabilize yourself by gently holding on to a table until you gain the fitness and confidence to do this exercise without any support. Complete 12 to 15 repetitions or as specified on your training plan.

c. Step-Up

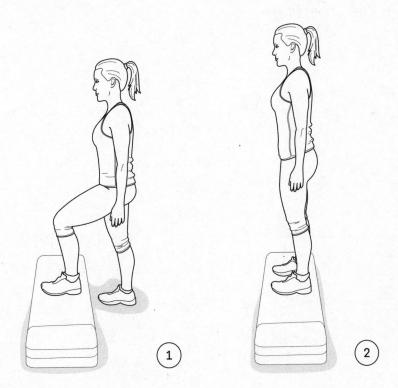

Place your left foot on a step. Keeping your toes pointing straight ahead, knee and hip aligned with your foot, step up, using the muscles in your left leg. Touch the step with your right foot. Pause only a moment and return to the starting position. Complete all repetitions working the left leg, then repeat with the right leg. Try to do 12 repetitions with each leg. Pause. Rest. And Repeat. Try for a total of 3 sets of 12 for each leg.

Wall Chest Press or Push-Up

a. Wall Chest Press

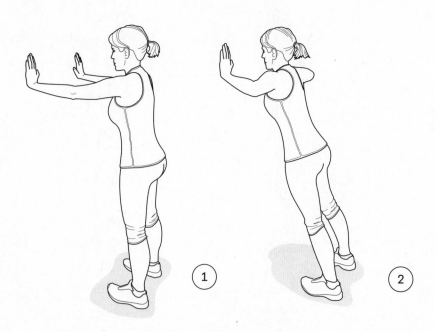

Begin by facing a wall, with your feet about 18 inches away from the wall. Place your hands on the wall, slightly wider than your shoulders, fingers pointing toward the ceiling or slightly in. Keep your body rigid during the movement by exhaling while contracting your abdominal and back muscles. With knees slightly bent, lower yourself toward the wall until your forearm and upper arm form a 90-degree angle, pause for a moment, and then push away from the wall. Your movements toward and away from the wall are to be done slowly, engaging your muscles to control the motion. As you gain fitness, you can move your body further from the wall or use the top of a counter for your pushing platform. Complete 12 to 15 repetitions or as specified on your training plan.

b. Push-Up

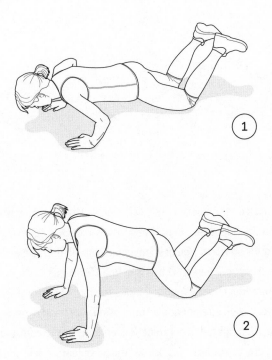

Begin by placing yourself facedown on the floor with your hands slightly wider than your shoulders—just like the beginning position for the Wall Chest Press. Fingers should be pointed forward or turned slightly in. Your floor contact points will be your hands and either your knees (an easier method) or your toes. With a rigid body, abdominals and back muscles contracted, push yourself away from the floor until your elbows are nearly locked—but don't lock them. Slowly lower your body back toward the floor in a controlled manner until the angle between the upper and lower arm is between 90 and 100 degrees. Pause for a moment before pushing back up again. Once again, the magic number is 1 set of 12 repetitions. After the first set, rest for a moment. Reposition yourself, and then do another 12. And then once again for 3 sets of 12.

Abdominal Exercises

a. Crunch

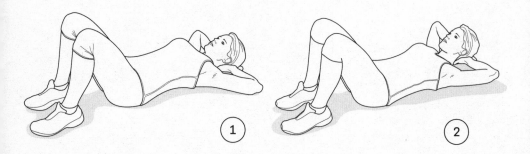

Lying on your back on the floor, bend your knees so that your feet rest comfortably on the floor. Make sure that your lower back is down and touching the floor. A slightly soft exercise or yoga mat is helpful for this exercise. Interlock your fingers and put your hands behind your head for support. Or you can cross your arms across your chest. When you move forward to perform the crunch motion, keep your neck straight and do not pull on your head or neck as you do the crunch. Exhale, then tighten or contract your abdominal muscles, bringing your bottom ribs up and toward your hip bones. Your shoulders, neck, and head follow, without pulling on your head. Don't apply pressure to your neck. The movement is complete when the tops of your shoulders have lifted off the floor and when your feet want to lift off the floor. Pause for a moment at this position, keeping your abdominal muscles contracted and your feet on the floor. Lower yourself slowly back down until you've returned to the original position. Don't cheat and just let go of your abdominal muscles, allowing your body to relax until it hits the floor. This is counterproductive. Maintain the crunch coming up and returning back down. That way you'll work the core and get a great result. Begin with 12 to 15 repetitions, or as many as you can do for the number of sets specified on your plan. As you gain fitness, it will become possible to complete 3 sets of 20 repetitions.

b. Opposite Hand to Knee Crunch

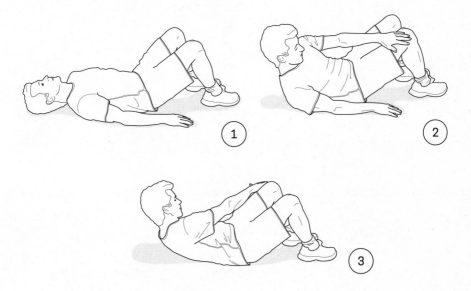

Lying on your back on the floor, bend your knees so your feet rest comfortably on the floor. Rest your arms on the floor with fingertips pointed toward your feet. Tighten or contract your abdominal muscles, bringing your bottom ribs toward your hip bones. Reach your left hand toward your right knee. The movement is complete when the left hand reaches the knee, or the left shoulder is off the floor and your feet want to come off the floor. Pause for a moment at this position, keeping your abdominal muscles contracted and your feet on the floor. Lower yourself slowly until you are back at the starting position. Again, don't just give up the crunch and relax your abdominal muscles, allowing your body to relax until it returns to the floor. Maximum result occurs from concentrated effort. Repeat the same motion, but this time with the right hand and left knee. Try for 3 sets of 12 each on each side. As you do one after the other, you sometimes feel a burning sensation as the muscles push to do the work. It only gets better as the entire abdominal region responds to the work.

c. Arm Pump Crunch

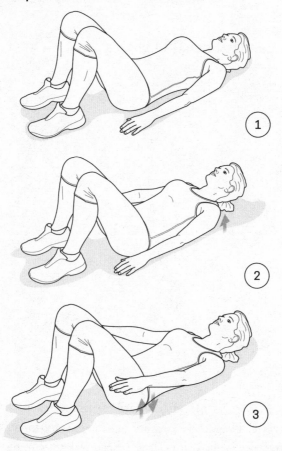

Lying on your back on the floor, bend your knees so your feet rest comfortably on the floor. Rest your arms on the floor with fingertips pointed toward your feet. Tighten or contract your abdominal muscles, bringing your bottom ribs toward your hip bones while lifting both hands off the floor about six inches and reaching toward your feet. With your abdominal wall contracted, pump your hands up and down slowly toward your feet for the count of five. Keep exhaling with each pump forward during the slow count. After the last pump, lower your shoulders slowly until you have returned to the starting position. As always, don't just give up the crunch and relax your abdominal muscles, allowing your body to relax until it returns to the floor. Try to do 3 sets of 5 pumps each. Maintain your form and remember to breathe and exhale, breathe and exhale.

Back Extension Exercises

a. Bent-Over Raise

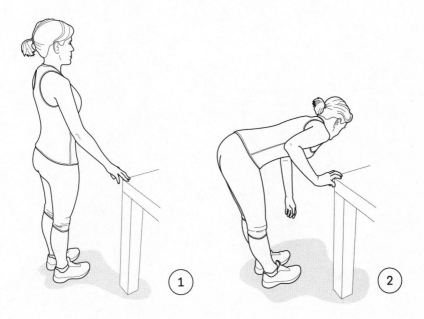

Standing next to your kitchen table, with a light touch, put your hand on the
table for support. Bending at the waist, lower your body until it is parallel with
the floor. Using the muscles in your back and butt (the gluteus maximus), slowly
raise yourself back to an upright position. As you gain fitness, use your arm for
assistance with this exercise less and less. Be careful in building these muscles.
Take your time and maintain your form. Complete 12 to 15 repetitions.

b. Superman (or Superwoman) Beginner

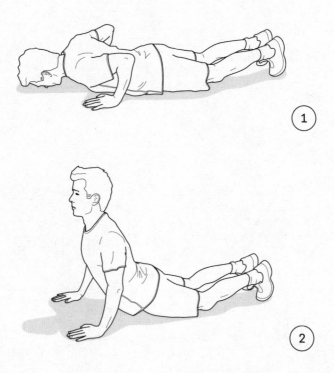

Lying facedown on a floor mat, place your arms forward, hands next to your armpits, fingers pointing forward. Using your back muscles, raise your upper chest off the ground, using as much arm strength as you need. Pause for a moment before lowering yourself back to the starting position with a controlled movement. During the exercise, your legs stay on the ground. Your neck remains aligned with your spine, maintaining its normal curvature. Complete 12 to 15 repetitions.

c. Superman (or Superwoman) with Extended Arms

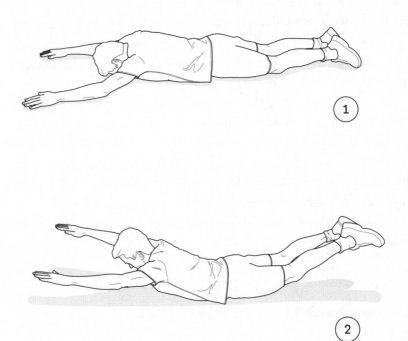

Lying facedown on the floor, extend your arms forward with your body in the longest position possible. Using your back muscles and butt muscles, raise your upper chest and feet off the ground. Imagine you are Superman or Superwoman, flying through the air. Pause for a moment before lowering yourself back to the starting position with a slow, controlled movement. During the exercise, your neck remains aligned with your spine, maintaining its normal curvature. Complete 12 to 15 repetitions.

GYM STRENGTH-TRAINING PROGRAM FOR THE LEVEL II TRAINING PLAN

You can continue the home program; however, progress will be limited by the weights available to you at home. For some people, maintaining a strength level at home is enough. Others will want to go to the gym to have access to more weights and a variety of exercise machines or other gym tools.

If you're doing strength workouts at the gym, and you're a newcomer, consult a qualified personal trainer to get you started and show you how to do each of these exercises. Here's a basic routine. Be sure to include a 5 to 10 minute warm-up prior to doing strength training. If you're a beginner, start with light weights (5 to 10 pounds) or no weight at all. That means you can use just your body weight.

To begin your gym strength-training program, complete 2 to 3 sets of 15 to 20 repetitions (reps) of five exercises:

1. Hip extension (choose one: squat, step-up, or leg press)

2. Supine dumbbell chest presses or push-ups

3. Seated row

4. Floor supine trunk flexion (also called abdominal curls or crunches) or exercise ball circles

5. Floor back extensions (also called Superman) or exercise ball back extensions

As you become more experienced at the gym, you can add more exercises. In all cases, begin with a weight that feels too easy. For a bigger, stronger person this "light" weight will be more than for a smaller or weaker person. It isn't about how much you lift compared to other people, rather your personal progress. Also, it is much easier to add more weight next time, rather than to begin with too much weight and hurt yourself.

1. Hip Extension Exercises

Choose one: Leg press machine, squat, step-up.

a. Squat with Barbells

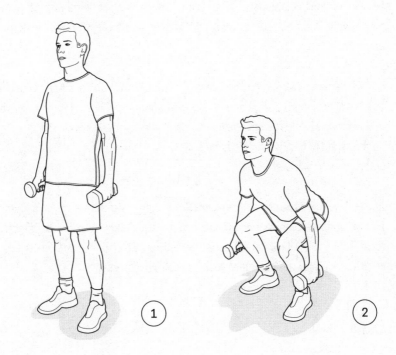

For this one, the movement is the same as the non-weighted version in the home strength-training workout on page 188. Just hold a weight in each hand that makes the squat movement slightly more difficult, but not too hard. You can also use the chair sit version on page 186 until you get used to the extra weight. Be sure to keep your feet pointed forward and shoulder-width apart. (As a variation, point your feet at a 45-degree angle and slightly wider than shoulder-width apart. Knees and upper legs point in the same direction as toes.)

In time, you might want to make the transition to squatting with a squat rack at the gym. Squat racks typically have mirrors, so you can watch to be certain your form stays good as you add weight. Before beginning with one of the squat bars (which weigh 35 or 45 pounds), search out a wooden handle at your gym. Most gyms have these around and they look similar to a broomstick. If your gym doesn't have a wooden or plastic stick, you might want to begin at home with a broom or mop handle. Practice squatting with the stick before trying the move with the squat bar.

Lift the bar or stick overhead and place it across your shoulders. Keep your hands comfortably placed on the bar, with elbows bent at roughly 90 degrees and palms facing forward. Hold the bar against your shoulders with straight wrists—not bent forward or backward. This hand position helps brace the bar in a straight line across your shoulders.

At all times, keep the correct form you used when you did unweighted squats. This includes keeping your chest pushed up and looking forward with a slightly tucked chin. Your elbows stay pushed behind you, which raises your shoulders to create a ledge for the bar out of your rear deltoid muscles.

b. Step-Up with Weights

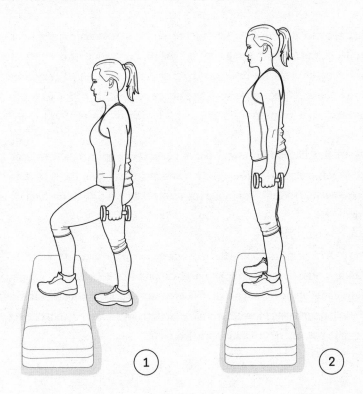

When first beginning, do the exercise with no weights. As you progress and gain strength, you can hold 5-pound dumbbells in each hand while doing the movement. Add weight over time as it feels comfortable. Place your left foot on a sturdy platform about mid-shin high, with your toes pointing straight ahead. Step up, using the muscles in your left leg, and touch the platform with your right foot. Pause for a brief moment, and then slowly return to the starting position. Keep your knees and feet pointed forward the entire time. Complete all repetitions working the left leg, and then repeat with the right leg.

c. Leg Press Machine

Adjust the seat so your knees are bent at roughly a 45-degree angle. Place your feet flat on the platform about shoulder-width apart with toes pointing forward or at a 45-degree angle pointing to the outside corners of the platform. Be careful not to place your feet too high on the platform so that your ankles are in front of your knee joints, or too low so that your heels hang off the platform.

Slowly press the platform away from you, until your legs are nearly straight, knees almost locked. Pause for as long as it takes you to say, "one-thousand-one" before lowering the platform. Keep your heels flat on the platform during this motion.

Using your muscles to control the movement, lower the platform until the platform is near the starting position—but don't let it touch down. This generally relaxes some of the muscles that should be working, lifts your butt off the seat pad, rocks your pelvis forward, and eliminates the normal curvature of the spine. Be sure to control the weight in both directions.

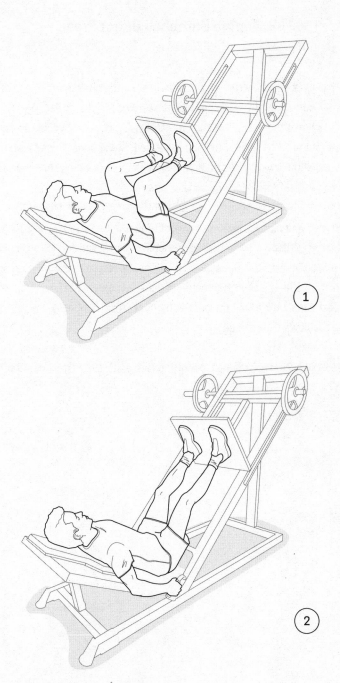

2. Supine Dumbbell Chest Press

Lie on your back on a bench with your back in a neutral position, one that allows the normal curvature of your spine to be present. Place your feet on the floor or on the bottom of the bench, whichever position is most comfortable. Holding a light weight in both hands with arms extended, keep hands aligned with the elbows and shoulder joints. Retract your shoulders—squeeze your shoulder blades together—before lowering the weight.

Leading with your elbows, lower the weight until your upper arm is parallel to the floor. Keep your elbows in line with your shoulder joints, and don't arch your back on the upward movement. Pause for a moment and return to the starting position by keeping your hands directly above your elbows throughout the movement. Don't let the dumbbells drift toward the center line of your body or away from your body on the upward movement.

You also have the option of doing push-ups. See page 191 in the home workout.

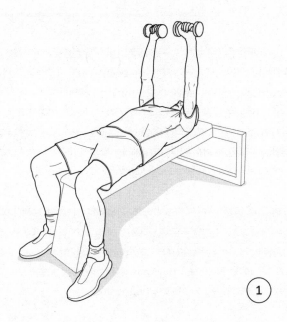

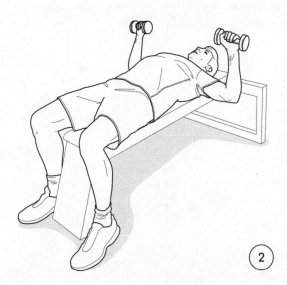

3. Seated Row

At many gyms there are different handles to choose from. Use a handle that puts your hands in a position similar to the one you use when holding on to bicycle handlebars. Seated, with your knees slightly flexed and torso and thighs forming close to a 90-degree angle, place your feet flat on the footplates. Looking forward, keep your head and neck upright. Your elbows should be nearly straight when handles are held at arm's length and there is tension in the cable. Your shoulder blades should be relaxed and separated (abducted).

Initiate the pull by retracting your shoulder blades together, then pulling the bar toward your chest, leading with your elbows. After a brief pause at the chest, return the handle to the starting position by moving first at your elbows, then shoulders. After your elbows are nearly straight, allow your shoulder blades to separate slightly, returning to the starting position.

Your back should remain still throughout the entire exercise, only flexing to return the bar to the floor when the exercise is complete. Keep your abdominal muscles contracted to stabilize your torso. Avoid flexing or bending at your waist and using your back to initiate the movement.

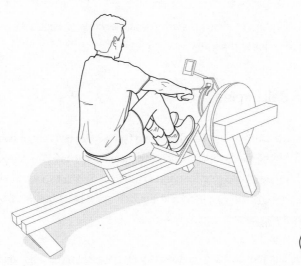

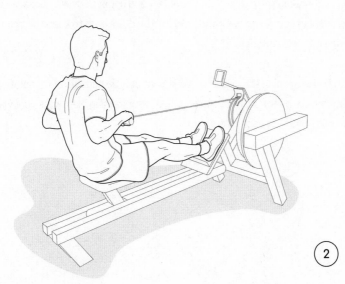

4. Abdominal Curls

See instructions in the home strength-training workout on page 192, or do exercise ball circles at the gym.

Exercise Ball Circles

Lie faceup on a gym exercise ball. These are typically big balls about two feet in diameter. Push the middle of your back into the exercise ball. With knees bent at roughly 90 degrees, keep your feet flat on the floor. Similar to abdominal curls, place your hands behind your head and supporting the head, but don't pull up and put stress on your neck.

Imagine pushing your belly button toward your spine, then your shoulders off the ball. Keeping your shoulders off the ball, trace a clockwise oval with the top of your head leading the movement. Shoulders and upper body will follow, as well. Keep pushing your lower back and belly button downward to keep the ball still through the entire motion.

When first beginning this exercise, you might only be capable of completing 5 circles in each direction. Over the course of your training plan, work your way to 3 sets of 20 circles in each direction.

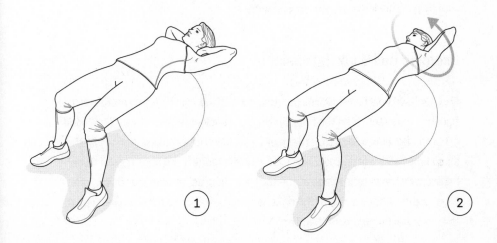

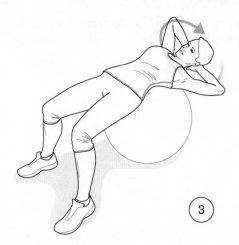

5. Floor Back Extensions (Superman)

See instructions in the home strength-training workout on page 197, or do exercise ball back extensions at your gym.

Exercise Ball Back Extensions

Lie facedown on a gym exercise ball. Begin with hands or fingertips resting on the floor and toes resting on the floor. Flexing your back muscles, lift your right hand off of the floor and reach toward the sky in a slow and controlled manner. At the same time you are lifting your hand, lift your left foot off the floor, reaching your heel toward the ceiling. Pause at the top for as long as it takes you to say, "one-thousand-one." Slowly return the right hand and left foot to the floor and repeat the movement with the left hand and right leg.

When first beginning this exercise, you will find balancing a challenge. The exercise helps you improve body balance and works the back muscles for a strong core. Also, when first beginning this exercise, you'll be capable of doing only 5 lifts for each arm and opposite leg. Over the course of your training plan, work your way to 3 sets of 10 lifts on each side.

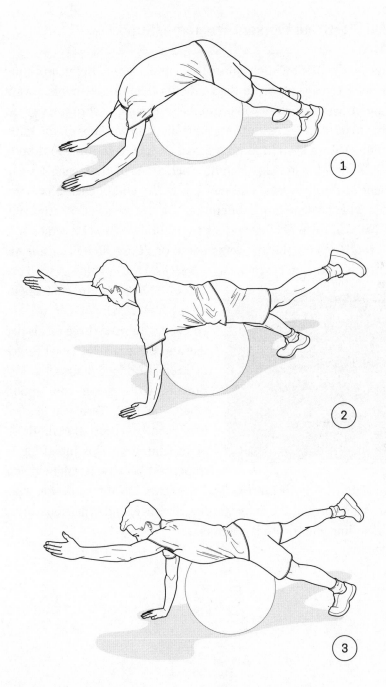

As You Start Your Workout Program . . .

The diet and nutrition information in Chapters Seven, Eight, and Nine is crucial for your success in the workouts. The two elements always operate in sync. So before you begin the workouts, be sure you've read the diet plans and are ready to start the diet and workout on the same schedule. Always keep in mind the goal—which is to train your body to stop being a fat-storing machine. Stick to the plan for each 4-week segment of the 12 weeks, and monitor at the end of each phase the ways in which it's making a difference. You can even check off weekly goals listed at the end of each week to celebrate your achievements.

If you happen to be an overachiever, don't overdo it. That means don't under-eat. Don't skip meals or snacks. Don't overexert with exercise. This program isn't about seeing how much you can torture yourself. You need three meals per day and three snacks. Don't forget to keep your food journal. Additionally, write down your mood when you ate. Were you happy, sad, mad, nervous, bored, tired, or just hungry? This mood log is important because it will help you notice patterns—both positive and negative. Do the same for your workouts, recording the activity, time, distance, and other measures, also including energy levels and mood.

> This program isn't about seeing how much you can torture yourself. You need three meals per day and three snacks.

ELEVEN

THE FAT-BURNING MACHINE WORKOUTS

Two Levels, Twelve Weeks Each

Whether you're starting this plan as a beginner or are more advanced, the best feeling in the world is to see yourself making progress from one level to the next. Each week of each plan builds on the previous week's work. Each day is a building block to better fitness. Once you have achieved a training intensity that suits your lifestyle, you can repeat weeks to maintain fitness. Or, you can look for new and more challenging ways to exceed your previous level of fitness. But once you're fit, you'll want to stay fit. Being a Fat-Burning Machine? It's fun!

In the 12-week plan, there are two levels with three phases each. Depending on your current level of fitness, you might want to enter the program at a later point rather than starting with Week 1. That's fine. There are guidelines in each phase that tell you if you should jump ahead. But still stay with a 12-week plan—so if you move forward, repeat the phase until you've done the program for 12 weeks.

LEVEL 1

Level I, Phase I

ATHLETE PROFILE: You are a beginner or currently a dormant athlete. You may not think of yourself as an athlete at all, but as human beings we are all athletes. Our bodies want to be active, in motion, and living life to the fullest.

You haven't exercised in quite some time. We're about to change that. We're going to work together to improve your health and fitness. You are a busy person and, for now, you don't want to go somewhere to exercise. You don't want to go to the gym, and your fitness program needs to be structured so you can exercise at home or at the office.

In this 4-week plan you will be walking or cycling only, with workout time ranging from 20 to 45 minutes. If you are already doing some limited jogging, you could use this plan as a jogging plan as well. Most of the workouts are intended to help you get your body in shape for higher loads. This means you won't be doing sprints or lung-busting long workouts in this phase. By being patient with your fitness, you stay healthy and avoid injury.

Exercise at least one day per week in the morning, shortly after waking up. Prior to this workout, do not eat anything and drink only water, tea, or coffee (no milk or sweetener of any kind in the coffee or tea). After this workout, eat your normal Fat-Burning Machine breakfast.

In the weekly charts, exercise days are shown as Monday, Wednesday, Friday, and Saturday. These days aren't cast in stone. You can move the exercise days to fit your personal schedule. If Tuesday, Thursday, Saturday, and Sunday works better for you, then use that routine instead of the one shown on the charts.

Lastly, some is better than none. If you get pinched for time and can't exercise for 30 minutes, do what you can. Even 10 minutes of exercise is better than none.

WEEK 1

MONDAY	TUESDAY	WEDNESDAY
Walk, cycle, or jog 20–30 min. FBE1* on a mostly flat course.	DAY OFF	Walk, cycle, or jog 20–30 min. FBE1. **MIRACLE INTERVALS:** After the first 10 min., gently increase pace to FBE2** for 10 steps or 10 pedal revolutions before returning to FBE1. Do this 4 times, with at least 2 min. between accelerations.

*FBE1 = Gentle, easy breathing
**FBE2 = More exertion, but enough to hold a conversation

Week 1 Goals:

1. Exercise 4 times this week. Feel free to switch days off with workout days, but try not to skip more than one day in a row.

2. Do at least 1 exercise session in the morning, before breakfast and on an empty stomach. (Water is fine.)

3. One exercise session this week includes Miracle Intervals, which are the shorter bursts at a higher exertion level—in this case, FBE2.

4. On non-exercise days, read the labels of 2 to 3 foods in your pantry, at the grocery store, or at a convenience store to learn how many grams of sugar are in one serving.

THURSDAY	FRIDAY	SATURDAY	SUNDAY
DAY OFF	Walk, cycle, or jog 20–30 min. FBE1 on a mostly flat course.	Walk, cycle, or jog 20–30 min. FBE1 on a mostly flat course.	DAY OFF

WEEK 2

MONDAY	TUESDAY	WEDNESDAY
Walk, cycle, or jog 20–30 min. FBE1* on a mostly flat course.	DAY OFF	Walk, cycle, or jog 20–30 min. FBE1. **MIRACLE INTERVALS:** After the first 10 min., gently increase pace to FBE2** for 10 steps or 10 pedal revolutions before returning to FBE1. Do this 4 times, with at least 2 min. between accelerations.

*FBE1 = Gentle, easy breathing
**FBE2 = More exertion, but enough to hold a conversation

Week 2 Goals:

1. Exercise 4 times this week. If possible, make one route different from last week. Feel free to switch days off with workout days, but try not to skip more than one day in a row.

2. Do at least 1 exercise session in the morning, before breakfast and on an empty stomach. (Water is fine.)

3. One exercise session this week includes Miracle Intervals, which are the shorter bursts at a higher exertion level—in this case, FBE2.

4. Remember to keep your food journal, writing down what foods you eat, when you eat them, and what your mood was before eating.

THURSDAY	FRIDAY	SATURDAY	SUNDAY
DAY OFF	Walk, cycle, or jog 20–30 min. FBE1 on a mostly flat course.	Walk, cycle, or jog 30–40 min. FBE1 and FBE2 on a mostly flat course. Don't try to maximize FBE2, just let it happen. For example, small hills will illicit FBE2. This is not a deliberate Miracle Interval, just an easy back-and-forth pace.	DAY OFF

WEEK 3

MONDAY	TUESDAY	WEDNESDAY
Walk, cycle, or jog 20–30 min. FBE1* on a mostly flat course.	DAY OFF	Walk, cycle, or jog 20–30 min. FBE1. **MIRACLE INTERVALS:** After the first 10 min., gently increase pace to FBE2** for 10 steps or 10 pedal revolutions before returning to FBE1. Do this up to 6 times, with at least 1.5 min. between accelerations.

*FBE1 = Gentle, easy breathing
**FBE2 = More exertion, but enough to hold a conversation

Week 3 Goals:

1. Exercise 4 times this week, with a course that includes gentle hills or inclines. Feel free to switch days off with workout days, but try not to skip more than one day in a row.

2. Do at least 1 and preferably 2 exercise sessions in the morning, before breakfast and on an empty stomach. (Water is fine.)

3. One exercise session this week includes Miracle Intervals, which are the shorter bursts at a higher exertion level—in this case, FBE2.

THURSDAY	FRIDAY	SATURDAY	SUNDAY
DAY OFF	Walk, cycle, or jog 20–30 min. FBE1 on a mostly flat course.	Walk, cycle, or jog 45 min. at FBE1 and FBE2 on a course with slight inclines. If you want to use stairs as your hills, that works. Just keep the uphill effort at FBE2. Downhill is FBE1. End with FBE1 intensity.	DAY OFF

WEEK 4

This is a recovery week. Exercise volume is intentionally reduced a bit. As you progress in your fitness program, these weeks become more important.

MONDAY	TUESDAY	WEDNESDAY
Walk, cycle, or jog 20 min. FBE1* on a mostly flat course.	DAY OFF	Walk, cycle, or jog 20–30 min. FBE1. **MIRACLE INTERVALS:** After the first 10 min., gently increase pace to FBE2** for 30 steps or 30 pedal revolutions before returning to FBE1. Do this up to 6 times, with at least 1.5 min. between accelerations.

*FBE1 = Gentle, easy breathing
**FBE2 = More exertion, but enough to hold a conversation

Week 4 Goals:

1. Exercise 3 times this week. Remember, this is a recovery week, with a lighter workout schedule. Feel free to switch days off with workout days, but try to schedule the workout days in a balanced fashion across the week.

2. Do at least 1 exercise session in the morning, before breakfast and on an empty stomach. (Water is fine.)

3. One exercise session this week includes Miracle Intervals, which are the shorter bursts at a higher exertion level—in this case, FBE2.

4. On non-exercise days, list non-food rewards for your success to be used this week and in the future. As you continue to succeed with the program, how will you recognize and celebrate success?

THURSDAY	FRIDAY	SATURDAY	SUNDAY
DAY OFF	DAY OFF	Walk, cycle, or jog 30 min. FBE1 and FBE2 on a course that has some gentle inclines.	DAY OFF

Level I, Phase II

ATHLETE PROFILE: This training block can follow Level I, Phase I, or if your fitness meets the following description, you can begin with this training block: You can walk, jog, or ride a bicycle (indoors or outside) 3 times per week for a minimum of 30 minutes at a time. Best scenario is if you are doing one longer workout each week that is around 45 minutes long. If you choose to start here, repeat the effort to match the 12-week program.

This 4-week plan will help you walk, jog/run, or ride a bicycle (inside or outdoors) for some 30 to 60 minutes. Additionally, this plan includes a home strength-training workout. As you've learned in Chapter Ten, strength training helps you build strength in muscles, tendons, and ligaments. This is not the kind of strength that a power lifter has; rather, it is strength that builds some functional muscles to help you burn fat. Also, you want the strength and balance to do everyday tasks for the rest of your life. Strength training can help you do just that.

Exercise at least one day per week in the morning, shortly after waking up. Prior to this workout, do not eat anything and drink only water, tea, or coffee. (No milk or sweetener of any kind in the coffee or tea.) After this workout, eat your normal Fat-Burning Machine breakfast.

GENERAL EXERCISE TIPS: Because you are already exercising, you know that it is important to have the proper footwear for your sport. If you're running and it has been many miles since you've gotten new running shoes, buy yourself a new pair. You have earned it, and it signals the new start.

Aim to stay close to the exercise guidelines. Each workout has a purpose, and it does you no good to exert yourself beyond the advised effort level. That is, don't make the sessions super hard. This is counterproductive to your goals of fat burning. Use the exercise intensity level guidelines in Chapter Ten as your guide.

In the weekly charts, exercise days are shown as Monday, Tuesday,

Wednesday, Thursday, and Saturday. Friday and Sunday are optional workouts. Do these if you have the time and energy for more than five days of structured exercise. You can move workouts around, but it is best to separate strength training by 48 hours. That means don't do strength training two days in a row.

A small amount of exercise is better than zero exercise. If you get pinched for time and can't exercise for 30 minutes, do what you can. Even 10 minutes of exercise is better than none.

This week introduces a strength workout twice a week. See Home Strength-Training Fat-Burning Exercises described in Chapter Ten, page 186.

WEEK 5

MONDAY	TUESDAY	WEDNESDAY
Walk, cycle, or jog 20–30 min. FBE1* to FBE2** on a mostly flat course.	**STRENGTH WORKOUT:** 15–20 min. Beginning conservatively, do 12 reps of each exercise.	Walk, cycle, or jog 30 min. FBE1 to FBE2. **MIRACLE INTERVALS:** After the first 10 min., include 4–6 reps of increasing your pace to FBE2 for roughly 10 sec. Go back to FBE1 for 1 min., 50 sec. between each acceleration.

*FBE1 = Gentle, easy breathing
**FBE2 = More exertion, but enough to hold a conversation

Week 5 Goals:

1. Exercise 5 times this week. Feel free to switch days off with workout days, but try not to skip more than one day in a row.

2. Strength-train twice this week. See the Home Strength-Training Fat-Burning Exercises in Chapter Ten.

3. Do at least 1 exercise session in the morning, before breakfast and on an empty stomach. (Water is fine.)

4. One exercise session this week includes Miracle Intervals, which are the shorter bursts at a higher exertion level—in this case, FBE2.

5. On non-exercise days, park in the space furthest out from your destination doorway (work, the grocery store, the mall).

THURSDAY	FRIDAY	SATURDAY	SUNDAY
STRENGTH WORKOUT: 15–20 min. Beginning conservatively, do 12 reps of each exercise.	DAY OFF	Walk, cycle, or jog 45 min. FBE1 to FBE2 on a rolling course (some hills or steps).	DAY OFF

WEEK 6

MONDAY	TUESDAY	WEDNESDAY
Walk, cycle, or jog 20–30 min. FBE1* to FBE2** on a mostly flat course.	**STRENGTH WORKOUT:** 15–20 min. Do 12–15 reps of each exercise.	Walk, cycle, or jog 30 min. FBE1 to FBE2. **MIRACLE INTERVALS:** After the first 10 min., include 4–6 reps of increasing your pace to FBE2 for roughly 20 sec. Go back to FBE1 for 1 min., 40 sec. between each acceleration.

*FBE1 = Gentle, easy breathing
**FBE2 = More exertion, but enough to hold a conversation

Week 6 Goals:

1. Exercise 5 times this week. Feel free to switch days off with workout days, but try not to skip more than one day in a row.

2. One exercise session this week includes Miracle Intervals, which are the shorter bursts at a higher exertion level—in this case, FBE2.

3. On one day, increase the inclines or hills. If you don't have hills where you live, use stairs for walking or jogging. On a bike, simulate hills by using a harder gear 5–6 times for 1–3 minutes, randomly during your ride.

4. Do at least 1 long workout of 45 minutes.

THURSDAY	FRIDAY	SATURDAY	SUNDAY
STRENGTH WORKOUT: 15–20 min. Do 12–15 reps of each exercise.	DAY OFF	Walk, cycle, or jog 45 min. FBE1 to FBE2 on a course that includes more hills than last week.	DAY OFF

WEEK 7

MONDAY	TUESDAY	WEDNESDAY
Walk, cycle, or jog 20–30 min. FBE1* to FBE2** on a mostly flat course.	**STRENGTH WORKOUT:** 15–20 min. Do 15–20 reps of each exercise.	Walk, cycle, or jog 30 min. FBE1 to FBE2. **MIRACLE INTERVALS:** After the first 10 min., include 4–6 reps of increasing your pace to FBE2 for roughly 30 sec. Go back to FBE1 for 1 min., 30 sec. between each acceleration.

*FBE1 = Gentle, easy breathing
**FBE2 = More exertion, but enough to hold a conversation

Week 7 Goals:

1. Exercise 5 times this week. Feel free to switch days off with workout days, but try not to skip more than one day in a row.

2. One exercise session this week includes Miracle Intervals, which are the shorter bursts at a higher exertion level—in this case, FBE2.

3. Do 1 long workout of at least 45 minutes. Whatever you did last week, make this week slightly more challenging. You can do longer hills, tougher hills, or increase your accumulated time in the hills.

4. Aim to try one fat-burning food that is new to you.

THURSDAY	FRIDAY	SATURDAY	SUNDAY
STRENGTH WORKOUT: 15–20 min. Do 15–20 reps of each exercise.	DAY OFF	Walk, cycle, or jog 45 min. FBE1 to FBE2 on a course that includes more hills.	DAY OFF

WEEK 8

This is a recovery week. Exercise volume is intentionally reduced a bit. This allows your body to rebuild and improve strength and endurance. Like work, recovery must be planned.

MONDAY	TUESDAY	WEDNESDAY
Walk, cycle, or jog 30 min. FBE1* on a mostly flat course.	**STRENGTH WORKOUT:** 15–20 min. Do 12–15 reps of each exercise.	Walk, cycle, or jog 30 minutes FBE1 to FBE2**. **MIRACLE INTERVALS:** After the first 10 min., include 4–6 reps of increasing your pace to FBE2 for roughly 30 sec. Go back to FBE1 for 1 min., 30 sec. between each acceleration.

*FBE1 = Gentle, easy breathing
**FBE2 = More exertion, but enough to hold a conversation

Week 8 Goals:

1. Exercise 4 or 5 times this week. The second strength workout is optional. This is a recovery week. Cutting back a bit this week allows your body to repair and get stronger.

2. Do at least 1 exercise session in the morning, before breakfast and on an empty stomach. (Water is fine.)

3. One exercise session this week includes Miracle Intervals, which are shorter bursts at a higher exertion level—in this case, FBE2.

4. On non-exercise days, list at least three successes. These can include items like consistent exercise, one workout before breakfast, one long workout, following fat-burner guidelines 80 percent of the time (or higher), etc. Recognize three steps you have taken toward better health.

THURSDAY	FRIDAY	SATURDAY	SUNDAY
STRENGTH WORKOUT: OPTIONAL. 15–20 min. Do 12–15 reps of each exercise.	DAY OFF	Walk, cycle, or jog 30 min. at FBE1 and FBE2 on a course that has some gentle hills.	DAY OFF

Level I, Phase III

ATHLETE PROFILE: This training block can follow Level I, Phase II, or if your fitness meets the description below, you can begin with this training block and double up. Before beginning Week 9, you can walk, jog, or ride a bicycle (indoors or outside) 3 times per week for a minimum of 30 minutes at time. Best scenario is if you are doing one longer workout each week that is around 45 minutes long.

This four-week plan will help you walk, jog/run, or ride a bicycle (inside or outdoors) for some 30 to 60 minutes. Additionally, this plan includes a home strength-training workout. (See Chapter Ten for instructions.)

Week 9 introduces a new level of Miracle Interval—the Miracle Tempo Interval—to indicate a higher level of performance. Miracle

Tempo Intervals are intervals or accumulated workout time at FBE3.

Aim to stay close to the exercise guidelines, especially the intensity levels. Use the exercise intensity level guidelines in the plan and Chapter Seven as your guide.

In the weekly charts, exercise days are shown as Monday, Tuesday, Wednesday, Thursday, and Saturday, although Friday can be optional. Do this if you have the time and energy for more than five days of structured exercise. You can move workouts around, but it is best to separate strength training by 48 hours. That means don't do strength training two days in a row.

A small amount of exercise is better than zero exercise. If you get pinched for time and can't exercise for 30 minutes, do what you can. Even 10 minutes of exercise is better than none.

WEEK 9

MONDAY	TUESDAY	WEDNESDAY
Walk, cycle, or jog 30 min. FBE1* to FBE2** on a mostly flat course.	**STRENGTH WORKOUT:** 15 to 20 min. Do 15–20 reps of each exercise. Repeat the full set for a second time.	Walk, cycle, or jog 30 min. FBE1 to FBE2. **MIRACLE INTERVALS:** After the first 10 min., include 4–6 reps of increasing your pace to FBE3*** for roughly 45 sec. Go back to FBE1 for 1 min., 15 sec. between each acceleration.

*FBE1 = Gentle, easy breathing
**FBE2 = More exertion, but enough to hold a conversation
***FBE3 = More labored breathing, spotted conversation

Week 9 Goals:

1. Exercise 6 times this week, choosing any day off that fits your schedule.

2. Strength-train 2 times this week, repeating the strength workout twice.

3. This week includes Miracle Intervals on 2 days, with an increase in intensity to FBE3.

4. One day is a long workout on a hilly course for 45 to 60 minutes.

THURSDAY	FRIDAY	SATURDAY	SUNDAY
STRENGTH WORKOUT: 15–20 min. Do 15–20 reps of each exercise. Repeat the full set for a second time.	**OPTIONAL WORKOUT:** Walk, cycle, or jog 30 min. FBE1 on a mostly flat course.	Walk, cycle, or jog 45–60 min. FBE1 to FBE3 on a hilly course. **MIRACLE TEMPO INTERVALS:** Aim to accumulate about 10 min. at FBE3 intensity over the course of your 45–60-minute activity.	DAY OFF

WEEK 10

MONDAY	TUESDAY	WEDNESDAY
Walk, cycle, or jog 30 min. FBE1* to FBE2** on a mostly flat course.	**STRENGTH WORKOUT:** 15–20 min. Do 15–20 reps of each exercise. Repeat the full set for a second time.	Walk, cycle, or jog 30 min. FBE1 to FBE2. **MIRACLE INTERVALS:** After the first 10 min., include 4 reps of increasing your pace to FBE3*** for 60 sec. Go back to FBE2 for 3 min. between each acceleration.

*FBE1 = Gentle, easy breathing
**FBE2 = More exertion, but enough to hold a conversation
***FBE3 = More labored breathing, spotted conversation

Week 10 Goals:

1. Exercise 6 times this week, choosing any day off that fits your schedule.

2. Strength-train 2 times this week, repeating the strength workout twice.

3. This week includes Miracle Intervals on 2 days, with an increase in intensity to FBE3.

4. One day is a long workout on a hilly course for 45 to 60 minutes.

THURSDAY	FRIDAY	SATURDAY	SUNDAY
STRENGTH WORKOUT: 15–20 min. Do 15–20 reps of each exercise. Repeat the full set for a second time.	**OPTIONAL WORKOUT:** Walk, cycle, or jog 30 min. FBE1 on a mostly flat course.	Walk, cycle, or jog 45–60 min. FBE1 to FBE3 on a hilly course. **MIRACLE TEMPO INTERVALS:** Aim to accumulate about 15–20 min. at FBE3 intensity.	DAY OFF

WEEK 11

MONDAY	TUESDAY	WEDNESDAY
Walk, cycle, or jog 30 min. FBE1* to FBE2** on a mostly flat course.	**STRENGTH WORKOUT:** 15–20 min. Do 15–20 reps of each exercise. Repeat the full set for a second time.	Walk, cycle, or jog 30 min. FBE1 to FBE2. **MIRACLE TEMPO INTERVALS:** After the first 10 min., include 4 reps of increasing your pace to FBE3*** for roughly 2 min. Go back to FBE2 for 2 min. between each acceleration.

*FBE1 = Gentle, easy breathing
**FBE2 = More exertion, but enough to hold a conversation
***FBE3 = More labored breathing, spotted conversation

Week 11 Goals:

1. Exercise 6 times this week, choosing any day off that fits your schedule.

2. Strength-train 2 times this week, repeating the strength workout twice.

3. This week includes Miracle Intervals on 2 days, with an increase in intensity to FBE3.

4. Your long workout is 60 minutes, with Miracle Intervals accumulating about 15 minutes at FBE3 intensity.

THURSDAY	FRIDAY	SATURDAY	SUNDAY
STRENGTH WORKOUT: 15–20 min. Do 15–20 reps of each exercise. Repeat the full set for a second time.	**OPTIONAL WORKOUT:** Walk, cycle, or jog 30 min. FBE1 on a mostly flat course.	Walk, cycle, or jog 60 min. FBE1 to FBE3 on a hilly course. **MIRACLE TEMPO INTERVALS:** Aim to accumulate about 15 min. at FBE3 intensity.	DAY OFF

WEEK 12

This is a recovery week. Exercise volume is intentionally reduced a bit. This allows your body to rebuild and improve strength and endurance. Like work, recovery must be planned.

MONDAY	TUESDAY	WEDNESDAY
Walk, cycle, or jog 30 min. FBE1* on a mostly flat course.	**STRENGTH WORKOUT:** 15–20 min. Do 15–20 reps of each exercise. Repeat the full set for a second time.	Walk, cycle, or jog 30 min. FBE1 to FBE2**. After the first 10 min., include 4–6 reps of increasing your pace to FBE2 for roughly 30 sec. Go back to FBE1 for 1 min., 30 sec. between each acceleration.

*FBE1 = Gentle, easy breathing
**FBE2 = More exertion, but enough to hold a conversation

Week 12 Goals:

1. Exercise 4 or 5 times this week, cutting exercise volume compared to the last three weeks. The second strength workout is optional. This is a recovery week. Cutting back a bit this week allows your body to repair and get stronger. Recovery is important, so don't do too much this week.

2. Do 1 exercise session is done in the morning, before breakfast and on an empty stomach. (Water is fine.)

3. Aim to reduce stress this week. Stress is an enemy of fat burning. For example, pause to take a few slow, deep breaths when you're feeling overwhelmed. Get a massage. Call a friend. And be sure to get eight hours of sleep.

THURSDAY	FRIDAY	SATURDAY	SUNDAY
STRENGTH WORKOUT: OPTIONAL: 15–20 min. Do 12–15 reps of each exercise.	DAY OFF	Walk, cycle, or jog 30 min. at FBE1 and FBE2 on course that has some gentle hills.	DAY OFF

LEVEL II

Level II, Phase I

ATHLETE PROFILE: This training block can follow Level I, Phase III, or if your fitness meets the description below, you can begin with this training block.

Before beginning Week 1, you can walk, run, or ride a bicycle (indoors or outside) 3 times per week for 30 to 45 minutes at a time. On at least one day of the week, you are doing a 45- to 60-minute workout. You are fit.

In addition to increasing your fat-burning ability, this four-week plan will help improve the average speed that you can walk, run, or ride a bicycle (inside or outdoors) at a given effort level. Notice that weekly workout time doesn't increase much at all—and you don't want it to. You are a person who has a certain weekly budget for workout time, and that is 30 to 45 minutes four days, 60 minutes on a fifth day, and sometimes an additional 30 minutes on a sixth day. You prefer one day off, or no planned exercise.

This plan includes a strength-training workout that needs to be done at a gym or utilizing home gym equipment. As you've learned in Chapter Ten, strength training helps you build strength in muscles, tendons, and ligaments. This is not the kind of strength that a power lifter has, rather it is strength that builds some functional muscles to help you burn fat. Also, you want the strength and balance to do everyday tasks for the rest of your life. Strength training can help you do just that.

You have the option of doing the strength workout at home or at the gym. If you are just beginning a strength-training program at the gym, consult with a personal trainer for at least one session to be sure you are using proper form. Using the right form when strength-training can prevent injuries.

Aim to stay close to the exercise guidelines. Each workout has a purpose, and you'll be most successful if you follow the routine as it's laid out. Overexertion is counterproductive to your goal of fat burning.

Use the exercise intensity level guidelines in the plan and Chapter Ten as your guide.

In the weekly charts, exercise days are shown as Monday, Tuesday, Wednesday, Thursday, and Saturday. Friday is an optional workout and Sunday is a day off. You can move workouts around, but it is best to separate strength training by 48 hours. That means don't do strength training two days in a row. For this plan, strength training at the gym (a home gym would work) is recommended. This is so you have access to a wide variety of weights and the option to use exercise machines. That written, you can maintain a certain level of strength by doing home exercises simply using body weight. For home strength trainers, you have the option to do the home strength-training exercises for 2–3 sets and 15–20 reps.

WEEK 1

MONDAY	TUESDAY	WEDNESDAY
Walk, cycle, or run for 30–45 min. FBE1* to FBE2** on a mostly flat course. **MIRACLE INTERVALS:** After the first 10 min., include 4–6 reps of increasing your pace to FBE3*** for roughly 10 sec. Go back to FBE1 for 1 min., 50 sec. between each acceleration.	**STRENGTH WORKOUT:** 30 min. Do 12–15 reps of each exercise, using a weight that feels light on each exercise. If you have been strength-training for a while, use a weight that feels "moderate." Repeat the full set for a second time. OPTIONAL: Repeat the full set for a third time. OPTIONAL: Gym strength-training program, 30 min., 12–15 reps of each exercise.	Walk, cycle, or run 30–45 min. FBE1 to FBE2. **MIRACLE TEMPO INTERVALS:** After the first 10 min., include 4–5 reps of increasing your pace to FBE3 for roughly 3 min. Go back to FBE1 for only 1 min. between each acceleration.

*FBE1 = Gentle, easy breathing
**FBE2 = More exertion, but enough to hold a conversation
***FBE3 = More labored breathing, spotted conversation
****FBE4 = Faster-paced, hard breathing

Week 1 Goals:

1. Exercise 5–6 times this week. The sixth workout is optional.

2. Using the home strength program, strength-train 2 times this week, using light (5- to 10-pound) weights. Repeat the routines twice. You have the option of repeating the strength exercises for a third time.

3. There are 3 Miracle Intervals this week, with accelerations to FBE3. One option is to begin with the gym strength-training program.

4. One day is a long workout on a hilly course for 60 minutes and it includes very fast, FBE4-level accelerations.

THURSDAY	FRIDAY	SATURDAY	SUNDAY
STRENGTH WORKOUT: 30 min. Do 12–15 reps of each exercise, using a weight that feels light on each exercise. If you have been strength-training for a while, use a weight that feels "moderate." Repeat the full set for a second time. OPTIONAL: Repeat the full set for a third time.	**OPTIONAL WORKOUT:** Walk, cycle, or run 30 min. FBE1 on a mostly flat course.	Walk, cycle, or run 60 min. FBE1 to FBE2 on a rolling to hilly course. **MIRACLE INTERVALS:** After the first 15–20 min., do 5–7 intervals of 20 sec. each at FBE4****. Take 4 min., 40 sec. at FBE1 between each Miracle Interval. Finish at FBE1 to total 60 min.	DAY OFF

WEEK 2

MONDAY	TUESDAY	WEDNESDAY
Walk, cycle, or run for 30–45 min. FBE1* to FBE2** on a mostly flat course. **MIRACLE INTERVALS:** After the first 10 min., include 4–6 reps of increasing your pace to FBE3*** for roughly 15 sec. Go back to FBE1 for 1 min., 45 sec. between each acceleration.	**STRENGTH WORKOUT:** 30 min. Do 12–15 reps of each exercise, using a weight that feels moderate on each exercise. Repeat the full set for a second time. OPTIONAL: Repeat the full set for a third time. OPTIONAL: Gym strength-training program, 30 min., 12–15 reps of each exercise.	Walk, cycle, or run 45 min. FBE1 to FBE2. **MIRACLE TEMPO INTERVALS:** After the first 10 min., include 4–5 reps of increasing your pace to FBE3 for roughly 4 min. Go back to FBE1 for only 1 min. between each acceleration.

*FBE1 = Gentle, easy breathing
**FBE2 = More exertion, but enough to hold a conversation
***FBE3 = More labored breathing, spotted conversation
****FBE4 = Faster-paced, hard breathing

Week 2 Goals:

1. Exercise 5–6 times this week. The sixth workout is optional.

2. Strength-train twice this week, using light (5- to 10-pound) weights. Repeat the routines twice. You have the option of repeating the strength exercises for a third time.

3. There are 3 Miracle Intervals this week, 2 with accelerations to FBE3. One day is a long workout on a hilly course for 60 minutes and it includes very fast, FBE4-level accelerations.

THURSDAY	FRIDAY	SATURDAY	SUNDAY
STRENGTH WORKOUT: 30 min. Do 12–15 reps of each exercise, using a weight that feels moderate on each exercise. Repeat the full set for a second time. OPTIONAL: Repeat the full set for a third time. OPTIONAL: Gym strength-training program, 30 min., 12–15 reps of each exercise.	**OPTIONAL WORKOUT:** Walk, cycle, or run 30 min. FBE1 on a mostly flat course.	Walk, cycle, or run 60 min. FBE1 to FBE2 on a rolling to hilly course. **MIRACLE INTERVALS:** After the first 15–20 min., do 5–7 intervals of 20 sec. each at FBE4****. Take 4 min., 40 sec. at FBE1 between each Miracle Interval. Finish with FBE1 to total 60 min.	DAY OFF

WEEK 3

MONDAY	TUESDAY	WEDNESDAY
Walk, cycle, or run for 30–45 min. FBE1* to FBE2** on a mostly flat course. **MIRACLE INTERVALS:** After the first 10 min., include 4–6 reps of increasing your pace to FBE3*** for roughly 20 sec. Go back to FBE1 for 1 min., 40 sec. between each acceleration.	**STRENGTH WORKOUT:** 30 min. Do 12–15 reps of each exercise, using a weight that feels moderate on each exercise. Repeat the full set for a second time. OPTIONAL: Repeat the full set for a third time. OPTIONAL: Gym strength-training program, 30 min., 12–15 reps of each exercise.	Walk, cycle, or run 45 min. FBE1 to FBE2. **MIRACLE TEMPO INTERVALS:** After the first 10 min., include 4–6 reps of increasing your pace to FBE3 for roughly 4 min. Go back to FBE1 for only 1 min. between each acceleration.

*FBE1 = Gentle, easy breathing
**FBE2 = More exertion, but enough to hold a conversation
***FBE3 = More labored breathing, spotted conversation
****FBE4 = Faster-paced, hard breathing

Week 3 Goals:

1. Exercise 5–6 times this week. The sixth workout is optional.

2. Strength-train twice this week, using light (5- to 10-pound) weights. Repeat the routines twice. You have the option of repeating the strength exercises for a third time.

3. There are 3 Miracle Intervals this week, 2 with accelerations to FBE3. One day is a long workout on a hilly course for 60 minutes and it includes very fast, FBE4-level accelerations.

THURSDAY	FRIDAY	SATURDAY	SUNDAY
STRENGTH WORKOUT: 30 min. Do 12–15 reps of each exercise, using a weight that feels moderate on each exercise. Repeat the full set for a second time. OPTIONAL: Repeat the full set for a third time. OPTIONAL: Gym strength-training program, 30 min., 12–15 reps of each exercise.	**OPTIONAL WORKOUT:** Walk, cycle, or run 30 min. FBE1 on a mostly flat course.	Walk, cycle, or run 60 min. FBE1 to FBE2 on a rolling to hilly course. **MIRACLE INTERVALS:** After the first 15–20 min., do 5–7 intervals of 20 sec. each at FBE4****. Take 4 min., 40 sec. at FBE1 between each Miracle Interval. Finish with FBE1 to total 60 min.	DAY OFF

WEEK 4

This is a recovery week. Exercise volume is intentionally reduced a bit. This allows your body to rebuild and improve strength and endurance. Like work, recovery must be planned.

MONDAY	TUESDAY	WEDNESDAY
Walk, cycle, or run 30 min. FBE1* on a mostly flat course. **MIRACLE INTERVALS:** You can include 4–5 reps of 10-step accelerations to FBE2** or FBE3*** as the mood strikes you to speed up a bit.	**STRENGTH WORKOUT:** 30 min. Do 12–15 reps of each exercise, using a weight that feels moderate on each exercise. Repeat the full set for a second time. OPTIONAL: Gym strength-training program, 30 min., 12–15 reps of each exercise.	Walk, cycle, or run 30 minutes FBE1 to FBE2. **MIRACLE INTERVALS:** After the first 10 min., include 4–6 reps of increasing your pace for roughly 30 sec. Go back to FBE1 for 1 min., 30 sec. between each acceleration.

*FBE1 = Gentle, easy breathing
**FBE2 = More exertion, but enough to hold a conversation
***FBE3 = More labored breathing, spotted conversation

Week 4 Goals:

1. Exercise 4–5 times this week, cutting exercise volume compared to the last three weeks. This is a recovery week. Cutting back a bit this week allows your body to repair and get stronger. Recovery is important, so don't do too much this week.

2. Do at least 2 workouts in the morning, before breakfast and on an empty stomach. (Water is fine.)

3. This week includes 2 very gentle Miracle Intervals.

4. For just one day, no eating after 7:00 p.m.

THURSDAY	FRIDAY	SATURDAY	SUNDAY
STRENGTH WORKOUT: OPTIONAL: 30 min. Do 12–15 reps of each exercise, using a weight that feels moderate on each exercise. OPTIONAL: Gym strength-training program, 30 min., 12–15 reps of each exercise.	DAY OFF	Walk, cycle, or run 30 min. FBE1 to FBE2 on a course that has some gentle hills.	DAY OFF

Level II, Phase II

Athlete Profile: This training block can follow Level II, Phase I, or if your fitness meets the description below, you can begin with this training block.

Before beginning Week 5, you can walk, run, or ride a bicycle (indoors or outside) 3 times per week for 45 to 60 minutes at time. One day of the week will be your long workout day. It can be walking, hiking, cycling, or running. Another option is to make this long day your team sport or game day. This means you can play tennis, softball, soccer, golf, or any other active sport you desire. If you have the energy and are motivated to exercise seven days per week, you can do the workout shown on Saturday on one weekend day and then do your team sport or game day on the other weekend day.

In addition to increasing your fat-burning ability, this 4-week plan is flexible for weekend activities such as hiking, golf, tennis, softball, soccer, and other fun. There are weekend workout options for those of you who love to move. Notice that Friday has an optional easy workout. Optional means that if you have the energy and desire, add that workout. If not, take a day of recovery.

This plan includes a strength-training workout that needs to be done at a gym or utilizing home gym equipment. As you've learned in the introduction to exercise and nutrition section in Chapter Seven, strength training helps you build strength in muscles, tendons, and ligaments. This is not the kind of strength that a power lifter has, rather it is strength that builds some functional muscles to help you burn fat. Also, you want the strength and balance to do everyday tasks for the rest of your life. Strength training builds that strength and balance. Notice that Tuesday is a light day for strength training and Thursday is a moderate day. On Thursday you will increase the weight just enough so it feels moderately challenging. Moderate doesn't mean pop-a-vein-in-your-forehead hard. An option to ease into moderate is to add small amounts of weight for each set. For example, if you use 5-pound weights, move up to 8 or 10 pounds. If you use 10-pound weights, move up to 12 pounds.

Aim to stay close to the exercise guidelines. Each workout has a purpose, and it does you no good to overexert. It will be counterproductive to your goals of fat burning. Use the exercise intensity level guidelines in the plan and Chapter Ten as your guide.

In the weekly charts, exercise days are shown as Monday, Tuesday, Wednesday, Thursday, and Saturday. Friday is an optional workout and Sunday is a day off. Add a Friday workout if you have the time and energy to do it. This may be the case for some weeks and not others.

Also know that you can move workouts around, but it is best to separate strength training by 48 hours. That means don't do strength training two days in a row.

WEEK 5

MONDAY	TUESDAY	WEDNESDAY
Walk or cycle 45–60 min. FBE1* to FBE2** on a mostly flat course. If you are running, aim for 30–45 min. **MIRACLE INTERVALS:** After the first 10 min., include 4–6 reps of increasing your pace to FBE3*** for roughly 20 sec. Go back to FBE1 for 1 min., 40 sec. between each acceleration.	**STRENGTH WORKOUT:** 30–45 min. Do 12–15 reps of each exercise using a weight that feels moderate on each exercise. You might be able to increase the weight on some exercises. Repeat the full set for a second time. OPTIONAL: Repeat the full set for a third time. OPTIONAL: Gym strength-training program, 30 min., 12–15 reps of each exercise.	Walk, cycle, or run 45–60 min. FBE1 to FBE2 on a flat to rolling course. You can use stairs or hill repeats if you don't live in a location with many hills. **MIRACLE INTERVALS:** After the first 15–20 min., do 5–7 intervals of 20 sec. each at FBE4****. Take 4 min., 40 sec. at FBE1 between each Miracle Interval. Finish with FBE1 to total 45–60 min.

*FBE1 = Gentle, easy breathing
**FBE2 = More exertion, but enough to hold a conversation
***FBE3 = More labored breathing, spotted conversation
****FBE4 = Faster-paced, hard breathing

Week 5 Goals:

1. Exercise 5–6 times this week. The sixth workout is optional.

2. Strength-train twice this week, using light (5- to 10-pound) weights. Repeat the routines twice. You have the option of repeating the strength exercises for a third time.

THURSDAY	FRIDAY	SATURDAY	SUNDAY
STRENGTH WORKOUT: 30–45 min. Do 12–15 reps of each exercise using a weight that feels moderate on each exercise. Repeat the full set for a second time. OPTIONAL: Repeat the full set for a third time. OPTIONAL: Gym strength-training program, 30 min., 12–15 reps of each exercise.	**OPTIONAL WORKOUT:** Walk, cycle, or run 30 min. FBE1 on a mostly flat course.	Walk, cycle, or run 60 minutes FBE1 to FBE3 on a rolling to hilly course. **MIRACLE INTERVALS:** After the first 15–20 min., do 5–7 intervals of 20 sec. each at FBE4. Take 4 min., 40 sec. at FBE1 between each Miracle Interval. Finish with FBE1 to total 60 min. OPTIONAL: Instead of the workout above, you can golf (walk the course) or play softball, soccer, tennis, or any other activity that you enjoy. Aim for intensities between FBE1 and FBE3.	DAY OFF

3. There are 3 workouts this week with Miracle Intervals, with accelerations to FBE4.

4. As an alternative to one workout, choose a sport like golf, tennis, soccer, softball, or basketball.

5. Notice that as you gain fitness, what felt "moderate" in the weight room in Week 1 now feels "light." You can adjust the weight in any week by adding a small amount until the load once again feels "moderate."

WEEK 6

MONDAY	TUESDAY	WEDNESDAY
Walk, cycle, or run 45–60 min. FBE1* to FBE2** on a mostly flat course. If you are running, aim for 30–45 min. **MIRACLE INTERVALS:** After the first 10 min., include 4–6 reps of increasing your pace to FBE3*** for roughly 30 sec. Go back to FBE1 for 1 min., 30 sec. between each acceleration.	**STRENGTH WORKOUT:** 30–45 min. Do 12–15 reps of each exercise using a weight that feels moderate on each exercise. Repeat the full set for a second time. OPTIONAL: Repeat the full set for a third time. OPTIONAL: Gym strength-training program, 30 min., 12–15 reps of each exercise.	Walk, cycle, or run 45–60 min. FBE1 to FBE2 on a flat to rolling course. You can use stairs or hill repeats if you don't live in a location with many hills. **MIRACLE INTERVALS:** After the first 15–20 min., do 5–7 intervals of 30 sec. each at FBE4****. Take 4 min., 40 sec. at FBE1 between each Miracle Interval. Finish with FBE1 to total 45–60 min.

*FBE1 = Gentle, easy breathing
**FBE2 = More exertion, but enough to hold a conversation
***FBE3 = More labored breathing, spotted conversation
****FBE4 = Faster-paced, hard breathing

Week 6 Goals:

1. Exercise 5–6 times this week. The sixth workout is optional.

2. Strength-train 2 times this week, using light (5- to 10-pound) weights. Repeat the routines twice. You have the option of repeating

THURSDAY	FRIDAY	SATURDAY	SUNDAY
STRENGTH WORKOUT: 30–45 min. Do 12–15 reps of each exercise using a slightly heavier weight. Repeat the full set for a second time. OPTIONAL: Repeat the full set for a third time. OPTIONAL: Gym strength-training program, 30 min., 12–15 reps of each exercise.	**OPTIONAL WORKOUT:** Walk, cycle, or run 30 min. FBE1 on a mostly flat course.	Walk, cycle, or run 60–75 min. FBE1 to FBE3 on a rolling to hilly course. **MIRACLE INTERVALS:** After the first 15–20 min., do 7-9 intervals of 40 sec. each at FBE4. Take 4 min., 40 sec. at FBE1 between each Miracle Interval. Finish with FBE1 to total 60–75 min. OPTIONAL: Instead of the workout above, you can golf (walk the course) or play softball, soccer, tennis, or any other activity that you enjoy. Aim for intensities between FBE1 and FBE3.	DAY OFF

the strength exercises for a third time. Use a slightly heavier weight on your second strength workout.

3. This week 3 workouts include Miracle Intervals.

4. As an alternative to one workout, choose an alternative sport like golf, tennis, soccer, softball, or basketball.

WEEK 7

MONDAY	TUESDAY	WEDNESDAY
Walk, cycle, or run 45–60 min. FBE1* to FBE2** on a mostly flat course. If you are running, aim for 30–45 min. **MIRACLE INTERVALS:** After the first 10 min., include 2–3 reps of increasing your pace to FBE3*** for roughly 30 sec. Go back to FBE1 for 1 min., 30 sec. between each acceleration. Then do 2–3 reps of increasing your pace to FBE3 for roughly 20 sec. Go back to FBE1 for 1 min., 40 sec. between each acceleration.	**STRENGTH WORKOUT:** 30–45 min. Do 12–15 reps of each exercise, using a weight that feels moderate on each exercise. Repeat the full set for a second time. OPTIONAL: Repeat the full set for a third time. OPTIONAL: Gym strength-training program, 30 min., 12–15 reps of each exercise.	Walk, cycle, or run 45–60 min. FBE1 to FBE2 on a flat to rolling course. You can use stairs or hill repeats if you don't live in a location with many hills. **MIRACLE INTERVALS:** After the first 15–20 min., do 5–7 intervals of 45 sec. each at FBE4****. Take 4 min., 15 sec. at FBE1 between each Miracle Interval. Finish with FBE1 to total 45–60 min.

*FBE1 = Gentle, easy breathing
**FBE2 = More exertion, but enough to hold a conversation
***FBE3 = More labored breathing, spotted conversation
****FBE4 = Faster-paced, hard breathing

Week 7 Goals:

1. Exercise 5–6 times this week. The sixth workout is optional.

2. Strength-train 2 times this week, using light (5- to 10-pound) weights. Repeat the routines twice. You have the option of repeating the strength exercises for a third time. Use a slightly heavier

THURSDAY	FRIDAY	SATURDAY	SUNDAY
STRENGTH WORKOUT: 30–45 min. Do 12–15 reps of each exercise, using a weight that feels moderate on each exercise. Can you increase the weight on any of the exercises? Repeat the full set for a second time. OPTIONAL: Repeat the full set for a third time. OPTIONAL: Gym strength-training program, 30 min., 12–15 reps of each exercise.	**OPTIONAL:** Walk, cycle, or run 30 minutes FBE1 on a mostly flat course.	Walk, cycle, or run 60–75 minutes FBE1 to FBE3 on a rolling to hilly course. **MIRACLE INTERVALS:** After the first 15–20 min., do 7–10 intervals of 1 min. each at FBE4. Take 4 min. at FBE1 between each Miracle Interval. OPTIONAL: Instead of the workout above, you can golf (walk the course) or play softball, soccer, tennis, or any other activity that you enjoy. Aim for intensities between FBE1 and FBE3.	DAY OFF

weight on your second strength workout. For example, go from 5 to 8 pounds, or 10 to 12 pounds.

3. This week 3 workouts include Miracle Intervals, with accelerations of FBE3 and FBE4.

4. As an alternative to one workout, choose an alternative sport like golf, tennis, soccer, softball, or basketball.

WEEK 8

This is a recovery week. Exercise volume is intentionally reduced a bit. This allows your body to rebuild and improve strength and endurance. Like work, recovery must be planned.

MONDAY	TUESDAY	WEDNESDAY
Walk, cycle, or run 30 min. FBE1* on a mostly flat course. **MIRACLE INTERVALS:** You can include 4–5 reps of 10-step accelerations as the mood strikes you to speed up a bit.	**STRENGTH WORKOUT:** 30 min. Do 12–15 reps of each exercise, using a weight that feels moderate on each exercise. OPTIONAL: Gym strength-training program, 30 min., 12–15 reps of each exercise.	Walk, cycle, or run 30 min. FBE1 to FBE2.** **MIRACLE INTERVALS:** After the first 10 min., include 4–6 reps of increasing your pace to FBE2 or FBE3*** for roughly 30 sec. Go back to FBE1 for 1 min., 30 sec. between each acceleration.

*FBE1 = Gentle, easy breathing
**FBE2 = More exertion, but enough to hold a conversation
***FBE3 = More labored breathing, spotted conversation
****FBE4 = Faster-paced, hard breathing

Week 8 Goals:

1. Exercise a maximum of 5 times this week, cutting exercise intensity compared to the last few weeks. Recovery is critical to becoming an efficient Fat-Burning Machine.

THURSDAY	FRIDAY	SATURDAY	SUNDAY
STRENGTH WORKOUT: OPTIONAL: Do 12–15 reps of each exercise using a weight that feels moderate on each exercise. OPTIONAL: Gym strength-training program, 30 min., 12–15 reps of each exercise.	DAY OFF	Walk, cycle, or run 45 min. FBE1 to FBE3 on a rolling to hilly course. **MIRACLE INTERVALS:** After the first 15–20 min., do 5–7 intervals of 1 min. each at FBE4****. Take 4 min. at FBE1 or FBE2 between each Miracle Interval. OPTIONAL: Instead of the workout above, you can golf (walk the course) or play softball, soccer, tennis, or any other activity that you enjoy. Aim for intensities between FBE1 and FBE3.	DAY OFF

2. Do at least 1 exercise session in the morning, before breakfast and on an empty stomach. (Water is fine.)

3. On one of your days off, investigate fat-burning foods you have yet to sample. Mix up your menus to keep eating enjoyable food and—of course—burning fat.

Level II, Phase III

ATHLETE PROFILE: This training block can follow Level II, Phase II, or if your fitness meets the description below, you can begin with this training block.

Before beginning Week 9, you can walk, run, or ride a bicycle (indoors or outside) 3 times per week for 45 to 60 minutes at time. One day of the week will be your long workout day. It can be walking, hiking, cycling, or running. Another option is to make this long day your team sport or game day. This means you can play tennis, softball, soccer, golf, or any other active sport you desire. If you have the energy and are motivated to exercise seven days per week, you can do the workout shown on Saturday on one weekend day and then do your team sport or game day on the other weekend day.

This phase includes variations on Miracle Intervals to indicate higher levels of activity. Miracle Tempo Intervals, as described earlier, are intervals or accumulated workout time at FBE3. Miracle Threshold Intervals are intervals or accumulated workout time at FBE4.

In addition to increasing your fat-burning ability, this 4-week plan is flexible for weekend activities such as hiking, golf, tennis, softball, soccer, and other fun. There are weekend workout options for those of you who love to move. Notice that Friday has an optional easy workout. Optional means that if you have the energy and desire, add that workout. If not, take a day of recovery.

This plan assumes you have been strength-training. Strength training goes into a maintenance mode in this training block with descending repetitions and increasing weights on one day per week.

If you are a seasoned fat-burner and you have reached your goals for health markers and weight, stay on track to maintain your success for a lifetime. If you are doing long weekend activities such as hiking or golf (walking a long course), be sure to carry a Fat-Burning Machine snack with you to keep the fire stoked in your fat-burning engine. Also, be sure to carry water and stay hydrated. If you find you often get behind on drinking, aim to drink twelve to twenty-four ounces per hour of activity. More when it is hot or you are thirsty. Less when it is cool outside.

Aim to stay close to the exercise guidelines—meaning, don't make the sessions excessively difficult. This is counterproductive to your goals of fat burning. Use the exercise intensity level guidelines in the plan and Chapter Ten as your guide.

In the weekly charts, exercise days are shown as Monday, Tuesday, Wednesday, Thursday, and Saturday. Friday is an optional workout and Sunday is a day off. Add a Friday workout if you have the time and energy to do it. This may be the case for some weeks and not others.

Remember, you can move workouts around. Aim to separate strength training by 48 hours. That means don't do strength training two days in a row.

WEEK 9

MONDAY	TUESDAY	WEDNESDAY
Walk, cycle, or run 45–60 min. FBE1* to FBE2** on a mostly flat course. If you are running, aim for 30–45 min. **MIRACLE INTERVALS:** After the first 10 min., include 4–6 reps of increasing your pace to FBE3*** for roughly 20 sec. Go back to FBE1 for 1 min., 40 sec. between each acceleration.	**STRENGTH WORKOUT:** 45 min. For each exercise, do the following: Begin with 1 set of 15 reps using a weight that feels light. Add a small amount of weight and do 10 more reps. For the third set, add a small amount of weight again and do only 8 reps. Repeat the process for each exercise.	Walk, cycle, or run 45–60 min. FBE1 to FBE2 on a flat to rolling course (or using stairs). **MIRACLE INTERVALS:** After the first 15–20 min., do 5–7 intervals of 30 sec. each at FBE4****. Take 4 min., 30 sec. at FBE1 between each Miracle Interval. Finish with FBE1 to total 45–60 min.

*FBE1 = Gentle, easy breathing
**FBE2 = More exertion, but enough to hold a conversation
***FBE3 = More labored breathing, spotted conversation
****FBE4 = Faster-paced, hard breathing

Week 9 Goals:

1. Exercise 5–6 times this week. The sixth workout is optional.

2. During this 4-week block, strength training is in maintenance mode. There is only 1 strength workout each week, and the routine is different.

THURSDAY	FRIDAY	SATURDAY	SUNDAY
Walk, cycle, or run 30–45 min. FBE1 to FBE2. **MIRACLE TEMPO OR THRESHOLD INTERVALS:** After the first 10 min. or so, include 4–5 reps of increasing your pace to FBE3 or FBE4 for roughly 3 min. Go back to FBE1 for only 1 min. between each acceleration.	**OPTIONAL WORKOUT:** Walk, cycle, or run 30 min. FBE1 on a mostly flat course.	Walk, cycle, or run 60 min. FBE1 to FBE4 on a rolling to hilly course. **MIRACLE INTERVALS:** After the first 15–20 min., do 5–7 intervals of 30 sec. each at FBE4. Take 4 min., 30 sec. at FBE1 between each Miracle Interval. Finish with FBE1 to total 45–60 min. OPTIONAL: Instead of the workout above, you can golf (walk the course) or play softball, soccer, tennis, or any other activity that you enjoy. Aim for intensities between FBE1 and FBE3.	DAY OFF

3. Up to 4 workouts this week include Miracle Intervals, with accelerations of FBE3 to FBE4.

4. As an alternative to one workout, choose an alternative sport like golf, tennis, soccer, softball, or basketball.

WEEK 10

MONDAY	TUESDAY	WEDNESDAY
Walk, cycle or run 45–60 min. FBE1* to FBE2** on a mostly flat course. If you are running, aim for 30–45 min. **MIRACLE INTERVALS:** After the first 10 min., include 4–6 reps of increasing your pace to FBE3*** for roughly 30 sec. Go back to FBE1 for 1 min., 30 sec. between each acceleration.	**STRENGTH WORKOUT:** 45 min. For each exercise, do the following: Begin with 1 set of 15 reps using a weight that feels light. Add a small amount of weight and do 10 more reps. For the third set, add a small amount of weight again and do only 8 reps. Repeat the process for each exercise.	Walk, cycle, or run 45–60 min. FBE1 to FBE2 on a flat to rolling course (or stairs). **MIRACLE INTERVALS:** After the first 15–20 min., do 5–7 intervals of 30 sec. each at FBE4****. Take 4 min., 30 sec. at FBE1 between each Miracle Interval. Finish with FBE1 to total 45–60 min.

*FBE1 = Gentle, easy breathing
**FBE2 = More exertion, but enough to hold a conversation
***FBE3 = More labored breathing, spotted conversation
****FBE4 = Faster-paced, hard breathing

Week 10 Goals:

1. Exercise 5–6 times this week. The sixth workout is optional.

2. During this 4-week block, strength training is in maintenance mode. There is only 1 strength workout each week, and the routine has changed.

THURSDAY	FRIDAY	SATURDAY	SUNDAY
Walk, cycle, or run 30–45 min. FBE1 to FBE2. **MIRACLE TEMPO OR THRESHOLD INTERVALS:** After the first 10 min., include 3–5 reps of increasing your pace to FBE3 or FBE4 for roughly 4 min. Go back to FBE1 for only 1 min. between each acceleration.	**OPTIONAL WORKOUT:** Walk, cycle, or run 30 min. FBE1 on a mostly flat course.	Walk, cycle, or run 90 min. FBE1 to FBE4 on a rolling to hilly course. If you're running, hold it to 60 min. **MIRACLE INTERVALS:** After the first 15–20 min., do 5–7 intervals of 1 min. each at FBE4. Take 4 min. at FBE1 to FBE2 between each Miracle Interval. Finish with FBE1 to FBE2 to total 60–90 min. OPTIONAL: Instead of the workout above, you can golf (walk the course) or play softball, soccer, tennis, or any other activity that you enjoy. Aim for intensities between FBE1 and FBE3.	DAY OFF

3. Up to 4 workouts this week include Miracle Intervals, with accelerations of FBE3 to FBE4.

4. As an alternative to one workout, choose an alternative sport like golf, tennis, soccer, softball, or basketball.

5. If you are exercising for 90 minutes or more, be sure to carry a fat-burner snack.

WEEK 11

MONDAY	TUESDAY	WEDNESDAY
Walk, cycle, or run 45–60 min. FBE1* to FBE2** on a mostly flat course. If you are running, aim for 30–45 min. **MIRACLE INTERVALS:** After the first 10 min., include 2–3 reps of increasing your pace to FBE3*** for 30 sec. Go back to FBE1 for 1 min., 30 sec. between each acceleration. Then do 2–3 reps of increasing your pace to FBE3 for 20 sec. Go back to FBE1 for 1 min., 40 sec. between each acceleration.	**STRENGTH WORKOUT:** 45 min. For each exercise, do the following: Begin with 1 set of 15 reps using a weight that feels light. Add a small amount of weight and do 10 more reps. For the third set, add a small amount of weight again and do only 8 reps. Repeat the process for each exercise.	Walk, cycle, or run 45–60 min. FBE1 to FBE2 on a flat to rolling course. **MIRACLE INTERVALS:** After the first 15–20 min., do 5–7 intervals of 30 sec. each at FBE4****. Take 4 min., 30 sec. at FBE1 between each Miracle Interval. Finish with FBE1 to total 45–60 min.

*FBE1 = Gentle, easy breathing
**FBE2 = More exertion, but enough to hold a conversation
***FBE3 = More labored breathing, spotted conversation
****FBE4 = Faster-paced, hard breathing

Week 11 Goals:

1. Exercise 5–6 times this week. The sixth workout is optional.

2. During this 4-week block, strength training is in maintenance mode. There is only 1 strength workout each week, and the process is different.

THURSDAY	FRIDAY	SATURDAY	SUNDAY
Walk, cycle, or run 30–45 min. FBE1 to FBE2. **MIRACLE INTERVALS:** After the first 10 min. or so, include 2–4 reps of increasing your pace to FBE3 or FBE4 for roughly 5 min. Go back to FBE1 for 2 min. between each acceleration.	**OPTIONAL WORKOUT:** Walk, cycle, or run 30 min. FBE1 on a mostly flat course.	Walk, cycle, or run 90–120 min. FBE1 to FBE4 on a rolling to hilly course. If you're running, hold it to 60 min. **MIRACLE INTERVALS:** After the first 15–20 min., do 5–7 intervals of 30 sec. each at FBE4. Take 4 min., 30 sec. at FBE1 between each Miracle Interval. Finish with FBE1. OPTIONAL: Instead of the workout above, you can golf (walk the course) or play softball, soccer, tennis, or any other activity that you enjoy. Aim for intensities between FBE1 and FBE3.	DAY OFF

3. Up to 4 workouts this week include Miracle Intervals, with accelerations of FBE3 to FBE4. There is 1 long workout day of 90–120 minutes (60 minutes if you're running).

4. As an alternative to one workout, choose a sport like golf, tennis, soccer, softball, or basketball.

5. If you are exercising for 90 minutes or more, be sure to carry a fat-burner snack.

WEEK 12

This is a recovery week. Exercise volume is intentionally reduced a bit. This allows your body to rebuild and improve strength and endurance. Like work, recovery must be planned.

MONDAY	TUESDAY	WEDNESDAY
Walk, cycle, or run 30 min. FBE1* on a mostly flat course. **MIRACLE INTERVALS:** You can include 4–5 reps of 10-step accelerations as the mood strikes you to speed up a bit.	**STRENGTH WORKOUT:** 45 min. For each exercise, do the following: Begin with 1 set of 15 reps using a weight that feels light. Add a small amount of weight and do 10 more reps. For the third set, add a small amount of weight again and do only 8 reps. Repeat the process for each exercise.	Walk, cycle, or run 30 min. FBE1 to FBE2**. After the first 10 min., include 4–6 reps of increasing your pace to FBE2 for 30 sec. Go back to FBE1 for 1 min., 30 sec. between each acceleration.

*FBE1 = Gentle, easy breathing
**FBE2 = More exertion, but enough to hold a conversation
***FBE3 = More labored breathing, spotted conversation
****FBE4 = Faster-paced, hard breathing

Week 12 Goals:

1. Exercise up to 5 times this week, cutting exercise volume compared to the last few weeks. Recovery is critical to becoming an efficient Fat-Burning Machine.

THURSDAY	FRIDAY	SATURDAY	SUNDAY
DAY OFF	**OPTIONAL WORKOUT:** Walk, cycle, or run 30 min. FBE1 on a mostly flat course.	Walk, cycle, or run 45 min. FBE1 to FBE3*** on a rolling to hilly course. **MIRACLE INTERVALS:** After the first 15–20 min., do 5–7 intervals of 30 sec. each at FBE4****. Take 4 min., 30 sec. at FBE1 between each Miracle Interval. Finish with FBE1. OPTIONAL: Instead of the workout above, you can golf (walk the course) or play softball, soccer, tennis, or any other activity that you enjoy. Aim for intensities between FBE1 and FBE3.	DAY OFF

2. Do at least 1 exercise session in the morning, before breakfast and on an empty stomach. (Water is fine.)

3. Look into scheduling a massage session for sport recovery or stress reduction.

Congratulations on completing a very challenging program. I remember the first time I accomplished Gale's combinations of Miracle Intervals and strength workouts. As my body found its rhythm, I was elated to feel better every day. My old plagues of exhaustion and hunger disappeared. I hope you've had that experience, too. Your new challenge is to find ways of incorporating exercise into your everyday life going forward. I've found that these plans stand the test of time; go back and redo the 4-week segments of your choice, creating your own schedule. Keep moving, and enjoy yourself!

TWELVE

BE A FAT-BURNING MACHINE ...FOR LIFE

Fitness Leads to Success and Happiness

OK. You made it to the last chapter. You have read my story, and hopefully you have started Gale's nutrition and fitness programs. Just the fact that you are here means that you are well on your way to becoming a Fat-Burning Machine. In just twelve quick weeks you will be able to go from fat to fit. How do I know? Because I did it myself.

But being a Fat-Burning Machine for life will require more than reading this book or going on the Fat-Burning Machine Diet. It requires a commitment to a Fat-Burning Machine lifestyle. I have now been a Fat-Burning Machine for nearly four years. There is not a day that goes by I don't think about it.

Marcela gave me the best piece of advice: "You need to love the food that you are eating. You cannot make the change unless you really embrace what you eat."

I can honestly say that I love the food that I eat. I look forward to my meals and don't feel that I am missing anything. I've had ups and downs over the years. I told you about when I was training for the New York City Marathon and some other races. But the hardest lesson

I learned was when I let the BLTs in my life. It is the small things that got me, not the large ones.

It was the bite of my son's chocolate cake, the lick of Marcela's ice cream (she does have one weak spot), or the taste of my daughter's sushi rolls. The BLTs add up, and they are not worth it. Eating is eating, and the impact that it has on my hormones is the same: A domino effect that I simply don't need.

Also, after training for the New York City Marathon for two straight years, I grew tired of running. So I decided to golf a summer. I played a lot of golf—maybe five or six rounds a week. I walked the course and I even carried my bag on some rounds, but it was just no substitute for the Miracle Intervals. My waist was getting larger, and I could feel my body composition change back a little. No one noticed except for me, but that was enough.

I decided to rededicate myself. I took out the BLTs, I put the Miracle Intervals back into my life, and I eliminated the word "just" from my vocabulary—as in "just" a slice of pizza or "just" half a bagel with lox. I didn't like the effect.

So here are my five tips for being a Fat-Burning Machine for life:

1. Own it. It took a lifetime to gain the weight, and it will take a lifetime commitment to keep it off. Affirm your commitment to be a Fat-Burning Machine and acknowledge your success. In my exercise room, I have a brag wall full of photos of all my races to remind me of all of the work I have put into getting to where I am.

2. Embrace it. Love the food. Look forward to your meals and challenge yourself to come up with more creative ways to create delicious dishes like the ones that we developed with our recipe team.

3. Enjoy it. I love when I can run in the park and listen to my music. Or when I can ski down a double black diamond or drive my tee shot 275 yards. Gale always says to me, "enjoy your fitness," and I do.

4. Protect it. Sometimes my friends and family will pressure me to change my nutrition or fitness habits. They will tell me to take a

break and enjoy myself. What are they talking about? I am having a blast.

5. Share it. I am not shy about telling people my story. I want them to know that I understand what they are going through and there is hope for them—a plan that can work. Share your story with others and they will benefit.

Being a Fat-Burning Machine for life means taking it one day at a time. You now have the tools and insights that you need to live the life that you want to live, to have the body that you want to have, and to achieve your goals.

I still have some open items on my bucket list . . . I am sure you do, too. Let's check this one off together.

FAT-BURNING MACHINE
Q & A

We've packed a lot of information and advice into this book, but we understand that this is new for you, and you might still have some questions. Here are the most common ones Gale and I have heard from our fat-burners.

How will I feel on the Fat-Burning Machine Diet?

As you change what you eat, you may have a dull headache. This is normal as your body adjusts to the new diet. Soon after, your body will go into a new gear. When I was heavier, I was plagued by constant colds and flu-like symptoms. These all disappeared. As I gained weight, I also developed acid reflux. After I ate, I would have intense pain in my throat. Ultimately, the acid reflux led to pneumonia twice in eighteen months from particles ending up in my lungs. Needless to say, I don't have acid reflux anymore.

How will this program change my energy level?

You will quickly feel a surge in energy levels and a desire to keep in motion. As soon as my body chemicals stabilized, the ups and downs of insulin and the carbohydrate crashes disappeared and my energy levels were much more consistent.

Will this program help me sleep better?

As a Fat-Burning Machine, you will find that your sleep will be more regular. The combination of change in nutrition and increased fitness will make you more relaxed. I found that I no longer felt tired during the day and could fall right asleep when I hit the pillow at night.

Will I still crave sugar?

Unfortunately, the cravings for sugar may never disappear. I find that the most difficult moment is after lunch and dinner. There is a ten-minute window where I crave something sweet—a piece of fruit or some sort of dessert. When I feel this happening, I usually try to eat some Greek yogurt or a high-fiber bar.

What if I am hungry between meals?

It is not good to be hungry between meals. In fact, becoming a Fat-Burning Machine means that you should never be hungry. I try to eat at least five times per day. I also try not to go into any meal hungry, particularly dinner. If I do, I am at risk for overeating. It is critical to minimize risk. If you are hungry between meals, eat fresh vegetables. Most grocery stores have small servings of already-cut vegetables available.

Will I be able to control what and when I eat?

Becoming a Fat-Burning Machine means that you are in control of what you eat. The whole idea is to fit this program into your life, not the other way around. I travel 50 percent of the time, which means that I am constantly eating out at restaurants, many of which I don't know. It really doesn't matter. I can always find things on the menu that will work for me. I am also much more aware of situations. I think through what my day will be like and plan my meals ahead so that I don't get into desperate situations with limited options. I will carry some staples with me just in case, including high-protein, low-sugar bars and sometimes a high-fiber bar. I will bring no-calorie flavored water with me on planes, and I love to carry baby carrots to munch on.

How easily can you do the activities you love?

Keeping energy levels high so that you can do the activities you love is the real benefit of being a Fat-Burning Machine. This program will enable you to perform better by helping you improve your fitness and performance.

Can you become a Fat-Burning Machine if you don't or can't exercise?

Of course you can. Becoming a Fat-Burning Machine means changing your eating habits so that you change from fat storing to fat burning. Syncing fitness to nutrition means finely tuning your Fat-Burning Machine. For people who don't or can't exercise, it just means that your Fat-Burning Machine will run slower. Over the time that I have been a Fat-Burning Machine, I was sometimes not able to exercise due to work constraints or injury. At these times, I found that as long as I watched what I ate, I could continue to maintain and even lose weight. It was just not as fast.

Is coffee allowed on the Fat-Burning Machine Diet?

Moderation is key. A cup of coffee in the morning might actually improve fat burning for a bit. But studies indicate that too much caffeine can actually have the opposite effect, causing negative symptoms, such as a speeding heart rate and an elevation in cortisol. Caffeine can also interfere with your sleep. Studies show that short sleepers have a higher incidence of obesity.

Can I use artificial sweeteners?

A limited amount of artificial sweetener is allowed, but use caution. Some studies show that when you consume an artificial sweetener, the effect mimics sugar. That is, your body releases insulin just as it would if you were eating sugar—thus impeding your fat-burning mechanism.

Can I use gels and sports drinks in training?

You only need to use gels in training in the few weeks or month before your major race, unless you are training over very long duration (two and a half to three hours). Recent sports nutrition evidence suggests that runners "train low, race high" when it comes to carbohydrates. That means you should train on water alone for runs of up to two hours, or longer if you have sufficiently adapted. Only introduce carbohydrates in the form of gels or sports drinks when you find that it is affecting training performance substantially. Only introduce carbohydrates in the form of chews, bars, or sports drinks when you find that it is affecting training performance substantially. There is some thought that plopping a big bolus of gel in your stomach is less effective at managing digestion during sports than initiating digestion by chewing. For this reason we prefer chews to gels. Also, take a hard look at your sports bars. Some have very, very high levels of sugar.

You can "train" your body to adapt to lower carbohydrate ingestion and to switch to a fat-burning metabolism quite effectively. However, if you have been relying on carbohydrates in training, it will take some time to get used to training without them. Gradually decrease the amount used and the frequency of use until you are just using them when absolutely necessary.

What is your opinion of fluid and carb intake for exercising?

Gale advises that, as a rule of thumb, you need to drink water during any run over one hour and most runs that are over two hours. Some people use gels for all runs, even those under an hour. This is unnecessary and, in fact, can be detrimental in that it does not allow your body to practice using fats as a fuel, a factor that can become vital during a marathon.

The ideal is to consume about twelve to twenty-four ounces of water per hour in training for runs over an hour and about twenty to thirty grams of carbohydrates (like a chew or bar) for runs over two hours—if needed. That is, if you find that you are unable to maintain your estimated run duration or intensity, you may need some carbohydrates or extra fluid (more likely). If you perform fine over longer runs with supplements, then only use them when you need to practice race conditions in the final few weeks before your major event.

Also, bear in mind that your nutrition needs for training vary from session to session, depending on the goal of the session. For example, for a high-intensity interval session, being well hydrated in advance (say two liters in the previous twenty-four hours) plus adequate carbohydrates (five grams per kilo of body weight per day) are vital, as it is hard to complete this type of session without adequate fuel and fluid, and it is hard to replace once the session has commenced. For longer runs with a goal of aerobic conditioning and fat-burning adaptation, it may be desirable to become carb depleted for adaptation purposes (as described above).

Can I eat unlimited vegetables at snacks and meals?

The short answer is yes, you can eat veggies all the time. The longer answer raises more questions. Are you eating all the time because you're hungry, bored, nervous, tired, sad, mad, or something else? If you're eating because you feel hungry—fine, eat veggies. If you're eating for another reason—drink a glass of water and go for a walk instead. In my experience, emotional eating is still emotional eating, no matter what the food. When I changed my diet I found myself eating bagfuls of baby carrots—to the point where I turned orange!

Can I have any drinks besides water?

You can have diet drinks, but try to consume them sparingly. It can be hard if you're a diet soda addict, like I was. Some people are sensitive to artificial sweeteners—that is, the drinks make them feel hungry. Also, some people believe they are similar to sugar in how they make the body behave. The only way to know for sure is to try them and see how you feel. Also be conscious of caffeine in popular diet drinks. Water with a twist of lemon or lime is good for some. There are some diet flavored waters on the market when you just need something different. Sometimes these products are too sweet. A trick is to fill half of a glass with the drink. Top it off with water (reducing the severe sweet taste) and then add ice to the glass.

Is there an easy way to measure quantities when I'm not in my kitchen?

Being aware of portion sizes is key. When you choose to eat a quarter cup of nuts, it needs to be a quarter of a cup and not an entire cup. Worse yet, no mindless eating out of a bag or jar. Serve yourself the portion you desire and put the rest of the food away. Here are some tips for measuring. Take a one-cup measuring utensil. Make a fist and compare your fist to the measuring cup. Is your fist the size of one cup, more like one and a half cups, or maybe more? This is how you will determine a one-cup portion size from here on out. You will "measure" based on the size of your fist. For example, give yourself a one-cup serving of steamed vegetables on your plate. Make a fist and see what the serving size looks like compared to your closed fist.

The next measure is for ounces of protein. There are a couple of ways to get three ounces of protein. One way is to use a mail scale or other digital scale to measure out a three-ounce portion of steak, fish, or poultry. A second way to get a three-ounce serving is to have the butcher measure it for you. Once you get the hamburger home, remove it from the package and make a hamburger patty out of it. How does this hamburger patty compare to the palm of your hand? Is three ounces of hamburger the same size as the palm of your hand, or is it less—or more? Is your palm the size of six ounces of protein? The palm of your hand is your protein measure.

Next, get a measuring-size tablespoon. Visually compare the volume of butter that would fit in a level (not heaping) tablespoon to your thumb. Is the serving of butter the size of your entire thumb or just the top of your thumb from the knuckle to the tip?

Finally, look at a one-ounce serving of cheese at the deli counter. Most of the time, a single slice of cheese, cut for sandwiches, is one ounce. If you would rather cut a one-by-one-inch block of cheese and compare it to your thumb size, this is another way to measure one ounce of cheese.

Now, only using your body, you can estimate portion sizes.

If you have additional questions that aren't addressed here, we encourage you to visit our website www.Fat-Burning-Machine.com, join our online Fat-Burning Machine community, and, if you like, sign up for our Fat-Burning Machine Online Subscription Nutrition and Training Program.

APPENDIX B

ACKNOWLEDGMENTS

MIKE BERLAND:

The origin of *Become a Fat-Burning Machine* is simple. It was my desire to share an amazing secret that I learned and wanted everyone else to know. I wanted to change the lives of millions of people like me, who had gained one to two pounds a year and just couldn't take it off—people who had tried every diet with fleeting success, and were about to give up and resign themselves to a life of just being fat.

After more than forty years struggling with my weight and countless diets, I had discovered the key to losing weight, keeping it off, and living an active life. I felt an overwhelming call to spread the word and not keep the secret to myself. I had become a Fat-Burning Machine, and I wanted everyone else to have the same opportunity to change their lives and become Fat-Burning Machines like me.

As with all dreams, I needed someone to believe in me—and that was my wife, Marcela. She always thought it was possible and supported me from the beginning. As I dramatically changed my eating habits, my exercise patterns, and my general outlook on life, she supported me 100 percent.

In fact, Marcela became my strongest advocate—preparing my breakfasts and dinners, shopping for food at the supermarket, and skipping the desserts she loved so much. Marcela gave up her home office so it could be converted into a gym. And when I spent most of the winter of 2015 at the kitchen table writing this book, she never questioned what I was doing. She knew it was a lifelong dream and a new beginning for me.

It was a much more humorous adventure with my kids. My son, Matthew, is six feet two and 180 pounds. I am five ten and, in the beginning, I weighed 245 pounds. We have the same shoe size. Matt likes to wear his clothes loose, and so from time to time he would borrow a shirt or a pair of pants (with a belt to cinch the waist). As I literally shrunk, our sizes became much closer, and some of my clothes became more desirable to him—and, because turnabout is fair play, some of his clothes suddenly became of interest to me. Now, when Marcela buys either one of us a shirt or sweater for a present, each of us has a right of first refusal. Lots of back-and-forth. I love it.

My daughter, Isabella, was with me from day one. She loved the food—hummus at dinner, salads for lunch, and egg white omelets in the morning. Isabella is a foodie and has a much more interesting palate than I do. While she was in high school, she would help with the shopping and show me how to make all the food more delicious. We would tease each other about certain foods: Isabella loves grapes and I would call them sugar cubes. I love Fage yogurt with Fiber One, which Isabella simply doesn't like. Both kids helped me kick my Diet Coke addiction.

Discovering, writing, and living the Fat-Burning Machine lifestyle takes a team. And I had the best. There were four characteristics that each person on my Fat-Burning Machine team had to possess:

1. Passion

2. Insatiable curiosity

3. Belief that anything is possible

4. Commitment

Dr. Laura Lefkowitz changed my life. She opened my eyes to the possibility of losing weight. From day one, she understood the helplessness that I felt. When she explained the chemistry of the body and how different foods worked, it opened my eyes. Once I knew the facts, I understood the consequences of eating different types of foods. It was easy from that point forward. The results spoke for themselves.

I was a fan of Gale Bernhardt for many years before I had the courage to send her an email. I followed Gale's online training programs to the point where I imagined I was her best customer. In person, she is even better. Gale is the quintessential geek turned coach. She is deeply analytical with a personality that makes you believe that anything is possible. Gale doesn't have the word "no" in her vocabulary. Her energy is contagious. We speak every Sunday night and it just makes the whole week so much better. She has given me the power of confidence.

When Judith Regan agreed to publish this book, I knew we were onto something. Judith has her finger on the pulse of society. She is a true visionary who sets the course for others to follow. And once she decided to publish this book, she has been behind me all the way. Judith has infused the process with enthusiasm, creativity, and publishing savvy.

From the beginning, Steve Gilbert has been my closest advisor on this project and a true friend. He recognized the potential of *Fat-Burning Machine*, but he also knew the watch-outs. He steadily guided Gale and I through the traps, and helped us realize our potential. Most importantly, he showed a deep interest in what we were trying to do and was willing to be one of our earliest participants. While he didn't agree with everything we proposed, he tried it out with great success.

On a dreary cold Sunday morning in April, Catherine Whitney came into my life. We sat at my wooden kitchen table, drank Pellegrino, and shared our ideas about becoming a Fat-Burning Machine. Catherine was key in helping us organize our thoughts and translate our ideas. She is insightful and clear-thinking. Catherine is unflappable and never sleeps—two characteristics that I love.

My own journey of being a Fat-Burning Machine took a whole reorientation to my body. I was deeply curious about how it worked and how I could change it. Many of the discoveries I am sharing in this book come from an amazing team that I assembled:

King Mike Keohane of Central Park was my running coach. When we started, I could barely run twelve-minute miles. As I am writing this, I am averaging 8:30s in my 10K runs. Mike was incredibly patient with me and just kept gradually speeding me up.

Matt Fraley was my strength coach. Matt exemplifies the best elements of a trainer—he is kind, demanding, and supportive. I left each workout stronger than I was when I started, and eagerly waiting for the next session.

Luis Mata was my integrated manual therapist, who kept my body functioning as I pushed it further than I ever thought possible. Keeping my body healthy as I trained to be an Ironman required rolling, massaging, and releasing. Luis inspired me to go harder with the confidence that my body would be intact when I finished.

Michelle Maturo taught me how to ride a bike for long road races. She inspired me to power up hills and keep up my cadence.

Finally, I want to acknowledge my mother, who was the first person I tried the Fat-Burning Machine program with. My mother has had weight issues for most of the past thirty years and it breaks my heart. She was fit for many years and then just started gaining weight and couldn't stop. At only sixty-seven years old, she had given up. I knew I could help her by sharing the Fat-Burning Machine program. The other option would be to get ready for increasing medical bills and loss of mobility.

My mother has already lost fifty-one pounds being a Fat-Burning Machine. She loves exercising and going to the gym. She sends me photos of what she is eating. After years of constant complaints about her ailments, our calls are great as she tells me about her beautiful garden, the bike rides she is taking, or how many laps she has swum in the pool that day.

I hope that all of you who are reading this book have the same experience that I have had. Becoming a Fat-Burning Machine changed my life. It can change yours, too.

GALE BERNHARDT:

I want to thank my mother, Margie O'Connell, and my father, George Klein, for their endless encouragement. During the production of this book, I lost my father, and I know he would have been proud. My entire family and extended family has always encouraged me to pursue my dreams. Though you are not all listed by name, know that I appreciate your endless support.

Special thanks to Mike for trusting me to solve a set of interwoven problems that others could not, and for pushing me to share the solutions with others.

To help us fine-tune the instructions in this book, and to give us more data on the benefits of this program, we recruited the first group of fat-burners. To all of you, we recognize your valuable contributions and feedback to make this book even better. Thank you, Rick Brent, Kay Collins, Deborah Croarkin, Peter Davis, Scott Ellis, Alisha Hall, Linda Kennedy, Ron Kennedy, Ted Mioduski, Danielle Polansky, Jan Reuss, Janet Saxon, and those who preferred to remain anonymous.

I'd also like to thank Dr. Stacy Sims for reviewing the protocol in the book and helping us explain some of the positive changes we were seeing in our first group of fat-burners. Her knowledge and experience regarding human performance across a wide range of individuals is invaluable.

Many thanks to our wonderful team of Fat-Burning Machine chefs who contributed recipes for the book: Danielle Polansky, Delbert Bernhardt, Linda Kennedy, Samantha Tritsch, Steve Gilbert, and Scott Ellis.

Thank you to Cathy Sloan for modeling proper strength-training form for the illustrations.

Thank you to Judith Regan and the Regan Arts staff for having the vision to turn the book into a piece of work that is better than we ever imagined.

Thank you to Catherine Whitney for helping two people blend voices and ideas into this helpful and informative book. A special acknowledgment to Scott Ellis, one of our original Fat-Burning Machines. A life was lost way to early; he lived life to the fullest and made the most of each day.

APPENDIX C

NOTES AND SOURCES

Nutrition and exercise science supports the tenets of the Fat-Burning Machine Diet. Here are key references.

EXERCISE-NUTRITION PHYSIOLOGY

Bernhardt G. *Training Plans for Cyclists* (Boulder, CO: VeloPress, 2009), 38–41.

Cameron-Smith D, Burke LM, Angus DJ, Tunstall RJ, Cox GR, Bonen A, Hawley JA, Hargreaves M. "A short-term, high-fat diet up-regulates lipid metabolism and gene expression in human skeletal muscle." *European Journal of Clinical Nutrition* (December 2009): 1404–10.

Cheng IS, Liao SF, Liu KL, Liu HY, Wu CL, Huang CY, Mallikarjuna K, Smith RW, Kuo CH. "Effect of dietary glycemic index on substrate transporter gene expression in human skeletal muscle after exercise." *American Journal of Clinical Nutrition* (August 2006): 354–60.

Friel J. *Fast After 50: How to Race Strong for the Rest of Your Life* (Boulder, CO: VeloPress, 2015), 239–241.

McArdle WD, Katch FI, Katch VL. *Exercise Physiology: Nutrition, Energy, and Human Performance*, Seventh Edition (Wolters, Kluwer, Lippincott, Williams & Wilkins, 2010), 420–30.

Mohlenkamp, et al. "Coronary atherosclerosis burden, but not transient troponin elevation, predicts long-term outcome in recreational marathon runners." *Cardiology* (January 2014): 1754–9.

Reaven G. "Insulin resistance and coronary heart disease in nondiabetic individuals." *Journal of Science and Medicine in Sport* (July 2010).

Schwartz, et al. "Study finds that long-term participation in marathon training/racing is paradoxically associated with increased coronary plaque volume." *Missouri Medicine* (March/April 2014).

Solomon TP, Haus JM, Cook MA, Flask CA, Kirwan JP, and the Obesity Society. "A low-glycemic diet lifestyle intervention improves fat utilization during exercise in older obese humans." *International Journal of Sports Medicine* (November 2014).

Stannard SR, Buckley AJ, Edge JA, Thompson MW. "Adaptations to skeletal muscle with endurance exercise training in the acutely fed versus overnight-fasted state." *Journal of Science and Medicine in Sport* (July 2010): 465–69.

Stevenson EJ, Williams C, Mash LE, Phillips B. "Influence of high-carbohydrate mixed meals with different glycemic indexes on substrate utilization during subsequent exercise in women." *Obesity* (November 2013): 2272–8.

Tunstall RJ, Mehan KA, Wadley GD, Collier GR, Bonen A, Hargreaves M, Cameron-Smith D. "Exercise training increases lipid metabolism gene expression in human skeletal muscle." *American Journal of Clinical Nutrition* (February 2003): 313–18.

Volek JS, Noakes T, Phinney SD. "Rethinking fat as a fuel for endurance exercise." *Journal of Science and Medicine in Sport* (August 2012): 1754–9.

MIRACLE INTERVALS

Creer AR, Ricard MD, Conlee RK, Hoyt GL, Parcell AC. "Neural, metabolic, and performance adaptations to four weeks of high-intensity sprint-interval training in trained cyclists." *European Journal of Sports Science* (February 2015): 13–20.

De Bock K, Derave W, Eijnde BO, Hesselink MK, Koninckx E, Rose AJ, Schrauwen P, Bonen A, Richter EA, Hespel P. "Effect of training in the fasted state on metabolic responses during exercise with carbohydrate intake." *Journal of Sports Science* (June 1997): 315–24.

Gonzalez JT, Stevenson EJ. "New perspectives on nutritional interventions to augment lipid utilization during exercise." *Applied Physiology, Nutrition, and Metabolism* (September 2014): 1050–7.

Lambert EV, Hawley JA, Goedecke J, Noakes TD, Dennis SC. "Nutritional strategies for promoting fat utilization and delaying the onset of fatigue during prolonged exercise." *The British Journal of Nutrition* (February 2012): 339–49.

Ortega JF, Fernández-Elías VE, Hamouti N, García-Pallarés J, Mora-Rodriguez R. "Higher insulin-sensitizing response after sprint interval compared to continuous exercise." *International Journal of Sports Medicine* (November 2014).

Van Proeyen K, Szlufcik K, Nielens H, Ramaekers M, Hespel P. "Beneficial metabolic adaptations due to endurance exercise training in the fasted state." *Journal of Physiology* (November 2010): 4289–302.

Van Proeyen K, Szlufcik K, Nielens H, Pelgrim K, Deldicque L, Hesselink M, Van Veldhoven PP, Hespel P. "Training in the fasted state improves glucose tolerance during fat-rich diet." *Journal of Applied Physiology* (January 2011): 236–45.

FAT-BURNING VS. FAT-STORING FOODS

Ahmed SH, Guillem K, Vandaele Y. *"Sugar addiction: pushing the drug-sugar analogy to the limit."* *International Journal of Sports Medicine* (January 2000): 1–12.

Ahmed SH, et al. *"Sugar addiction: pushing the drug-sugar analogy to the limit."* *Current Opinion in Clinical Nutrition Metabolism Care* (July 2013): 434–9

Centers for Disease Control and Prevention. "Trans Fat." Accessed July 22, 2015. www.cdc.gov/nutrition/everyone/basics/fat/transfat.html

Harvard School of Public Health. "Carbohydrates and Blood Sugar." Accessed July 22, 2015. www.hsph.harvard.edu/nutritionsource/carbohydrates/carbohydrates-and-blood-sugar

Kilding AE, Overton C, Gleave J. "Effects of caffeine, sodium bicarbonate, and their combined ingestion on high-intensity cycling performance." *Journal of Sports Medicine and Physical Fitness* (September 2008): 320–5.

Malaisse W, Vanonderbergen A, Louchami K, Jijakli H, Francine Malaisse-Lagae F. "Effects of artificial sweeteners on insulin release and cationic fluxes in rat pancreatic islets." *Cellular Signalling*, Volume 10, Issue 10 (November 1998): 727–33.

Marieb EN. *Human Anatomy and Physiology*, Third Edition (Benjamin/Cummings Publishing Company: 1995), 43–45.

McNaughton LR, Lovell RJ, Siegler JC, Midgley AW, Sandstrom M, Bentley DJ. "The effects of caffeine ingestion on time trial cycling performance." *Hepatology* (April 2014): 1235–8.

National Heart, Lung, and Blood Institute Obesity Research. "NHLBI Obesity Research." Accessed July 22, 2015. www.nhlbi.nih.gov/research/resources/obesity

Schulte EM, Avena NM, Gearhardt AN. "Which foods may be addictive? The roles of processing, fat content, and glycemic load." *Journal of Primary Care and Community Health* (October 2014): 263–70.

Schulte EM, et al. "Which foods may be addictive? The roles of processing, fat content, and glycemic load." *PLoS One* (February 2015.)

Swarna Nantha Y, "Addiction to sugar and its link to health morbidity: a primer for newer primary care and public health initiatives in Malaysia." *Journal of Primary Care and Community Health* (October 2014): 263–70.

Volek JS, Phinney SD. "The Sad Saga of Saturated Fat" *Art and Science of Low Carb* (May 14, 2013) www.artandscienceoflowcarb.com/the-sad-saga-of-saturated-fat

INDEX

Note: Page numbers in italics indicate figure; page numbers followed by "t" indicate tables.